SUPPLEMENTS
FOR
SUPERHEALTH

What to take and
when to take them

Patrick Holford

PIATKUS

Other books by Patrick Holford

The Optimum Nutrition Bible

100% Health

The Optimum Nutrition Cookbook (with Judy Ridgway)

Beat Stress and Fatigue

Boost Your Immune System (with Jennifer Meek)

Say No to Arthritis

Say No to Cancer

Say No to Heart Disease

Balancing Hormones Naturally (with Kate Neil)

Improve Your Digestion

The 30-Day Fatburner Diet

The Whole Health Manual

Mental Health and Illness – The Nutrition Connection

© 2000 Patrick Holford

First published in 2000 by
Judy Piatkus (Publishers) Ltd
5 Windmill Street, London W1P 1HF
E-mail: info@piatkus.co.uk

For the latest news and information on all our titles
visit our new website at www.piatkus.co.uk

The moral rights of the author have been asserted

A catalogue record for this book is available from the British Library

ISBN 0-7499-1963-9

Designed by Paul Saunders
Typeset by Action Publishing Technology, Gloucester
Printed and bound in Great Britain by
Mackays of Chatham PLC

Contents

PART 3

ACKNOWLEDGEMENTS

I am most grateful to the following people for helping me collate and edit the information for this book: Natalie Savona, Sharon Kaye, Kelly Davis, Rachel Winning and Jennifer Meek for help with immune boosting nutrients. Also, I'd like to thank Piatkus for their excellent support.

GUIDE TO ABBREVIATIONS AND MEASURES

1 gram (g) = 1000 milligrams (mg) = 1,000,000 micrograms (mcg or μg)

Most vitamins are measured in milligrams or micrograms. Vitamins A, D and E are also measured in International Units (iu), a measurement designed to standardise the various forms of these vitamins that have different potencies.

1mcg of retinol (1mcg RE)	=	3.3iu of vitamin A
1mcg RE of beta carotene	=	6mcg of beta carotene
100iu of vitamin D	=	2.5mcg
100iu of vitamin E	=	67mg

REFERENCES AND FURTHER SOURCES OF INFORMATION

Hundreds of references from respected scientific literature have been used in writing this book. Details of specific studies referred to are listed on pages 170–7. Other supporting research for statements made is available from the Lamberts Library at the Institute for Optimum Nutrition (ION – see page 180), whose members are free to visit and study there. ION also offers information services, including literature and library search facilities, for readers who would like to access scientific literature on specific subjects. On pages 178–9, you will find a list of the best books to read to follow up the information in this book.

How to Use This Book

This book gives you all the information you need in order to sensibly supplement your diet for superhealth. With so many nutritional supplements to choose from, and new nutrients being discovered all the time, this is a complex subject but I have tried to simplify it by emphasising the main principles.

◆ KEY NUTRIENTS

Firstly, I have focused only on key nutrients – the ones that have the most substantial body of research to support their claims. (This does not mean that nutrients or supplements not mentioned don't also have benefits.)

◆ OPTIMUM AMOUNTS

Every section on a nutrient ends with an 'Optimum intake'. This is an estimate of what the average person may need for superhealth on a daily basis. In reality, of course, everyone is different and has somewhat different nutritional needs. The 'From diet' amount is an estimate of what you might achieve from a reasonably healthy diet, having read my book *The Optimum Nutrition Bible*, or having followed the recipes in *The Optimum Nutrition Cookbook*. The 'From supplements' amount equals the difference between the 'From diet' amount and the 'Optimum intake'. This tells you roughly what level of each nutrient you are likely to benefit from supplementing.

◆ OVERLAP

Nutrients are often found in many different supplements. For example, vitamin A is found in many multivitamins, antioxidant formulae and immune formulae. Part 3 explains how to combine supplements to gain the best overall balance. The important point is not to exceed the levels given in the chart on page xx.

If you're new to the world of nutritional supplements, don't worry. This book tells you what you need to know and what you need to supplement for superhealth. The effects of taking the right supplements can often be felt within a month, in terms of increased energy, mental clarity and stress resistance. After three months you may notice an improvement in your skin, hair and nails. The long-term effects, however, are the most exciting. Optimum nutrition (which means both eating the right diet and taking supplements) is the most effective way to prevent a myriad of common Western diseases, including heart disease, cancer, arthritis, diabetes and Alzheimer's. It is also the most effective way to slow down the ageing process. In short, if you want a long and healthy life take supplements.

part 1

chapter 1

Who Needs
Supplements?

◆ THE MYTH OF THE WELL-BALANCED DIET

You know the oft-quoted saying, 'As long as you eat a well-balanced diet you get all the vitamins you need'? This is actually the greatest lie in nutrition today. Why? Because every single survey conducted in Britain over the last decade shows that the British population (even those who say they eat a balanced diet) fail to eat anything like the Recommended Daily Amounts (RDAs) of vitamins and minerals.[1]

The shortfall is not minor. For example, the average daily intake of zinc in the UK population is 7.6mg – half the RDA of 15mg. With the possible exception of niacin (vitamin B3) and calcium, the average intakes of all remaining nutrients fail to meet the RDA levels, designed to protect against vitamin deficiency disease. If most people fail to take in these basic levels of the majority of nutrients, what are the chances that your diet is giving you at least the RDA of every single nutrient? Probably less than one in a hundred (see Figure 1).

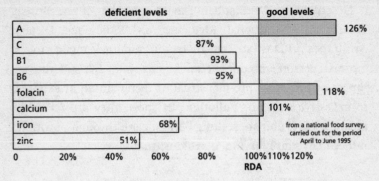

Figure 1 – Average intake as a percentage of the EU RDA

◆ RIDICULOUS DIETARY ARBITRARIES

RDA levels are set by government-appointed groups of scientists, based on how much of a nutrient is needed to prevent serious vitamin deficiency diseases such as scurvy (vitamin C), beriberi (B1) or pellagra (B3). Surprisingly, health authorities cannot agree on how much this amount should be, as shown by the fact that RDAs vary by as much as ten times from one country to another.

Many nutrition experts now consider RDAs to be considerably below the level of intake consistent with optimal health. Over the past 20 years RDA levels have gradually drifted upwards as the importance of optimum nutrition has increasingly been recognised. The National Food Council, which sets the RDAs for the USA, says that RDA levels are 'not necessarily optimal'. The EC's Scientific Committee for Food recognises that 'some nutrients have extra health benefits at intakes very much higher than those needed to prevent recognised deficiency signs. The Committee considers the evidence insufficient at present to justify making quantitative recommendations in this regard, but the results are awaited with interest.'

Described by Dr Stephen Davies, founder of the British Society for Nutritional Medicine, as 'Ridiculous Dietary Arbitraries', RDAs are, at best, the minimal intake for a 'normal' person who doesn't smoke or drink, isn't suffering an illness or infection, pre-menstrual or menopausal, or exposed to excessive stress or pollution. In short, they are relatively meaningless if you are seeking better health through nutrition, rather than simply trying to avoid getting scurvy.

◆ WHY RDAs ARE NOT ENOUGH

Consider vitamins C and E, which have been extensively researched due to their role in the prevention of cancers and cardiovascular disease. Numerous studies have indicated that an intake of vitamin E above 400iu offers maximum protection against these types of illness. In a Cambridge University study in which 2000 heart disease patients were given 400iu of vitamin E there was a massive 75 per cent reduction in the incidence of heart attack when compared to the placebo group.[2] The RDA for vitamin E is only 10iu.

Likewise, the protective role of vitamin C against various cancers, cardiovascular disease and the common cold only becomes significant above 400–1000mg a day. For example, a professor of medicine, Dr Harry Hemila, examined all research trials investigating the effects of vitamin C on the common cold. He selected only those controlled studies in which 1000mg or more of vitamin C had been given, and had been compared to a placebo. In 37 out of 38 trials, he concluded that supplementing 1000mg (20 times the RDA) had a protective effect.[3]

In a large survey in the US, analysed by Dr Enstrom and Dr Pauling, significant reductions in overall mortality and mortality from cancer and cardiovascular disease were reported in those who supplemented vitamins E and C.[4] Using the Cornell Medical Index, which is a general health questionnaire, Dr Cheraskin found the highest health rating among doctors whose vitamin C intake was above 400mg a day.[5] Yet the RDA for vitamin C is only 60mg – the equivalent of an orange a day.

From the scientific literature it would seem that if you want average poor health all you need is the RDA levels. However, for optimal health, maximum efficiency and freedom from disease, you need much higher intakes of essential nutrients. If you consider health as an abundance of well-being (not merely the absence of disease) then 'deficiency' is a lack of efficiency, such as having an immune system that is unable to combat a cold effectively. Well-being is measured by symptoms of deficiency (lack of energy, poor skin, emotional instability, frequent infections, etc) and by blood tests. We have measured the former at the Institute for Optimum Nutrition over a decade.[6] The results show that the 'average' person has 28 symptoms associated with deficiency, and after six months of adding vitamin and mineral supplements to their 'well-balanced' diet, the average number of symptoms drops to four. For example, in one survey 79 per cent of participants experienced a definite improvement in energy. Blood testing at a leading UK laboratory found that more than seven in ten people were borderline or severely deficient in B vitamins using accepted criteria for functional vitamin tests.[7]

The fact is that the RDAs are simply not enough for optimal health. This was shown conclusively by a 15-year study, involving 13,500 people, which established optimal nutrient intakes based on the results of blood tests, physical, dental and eye examinations and symptom questionnaires.[8] The conclusion was that optimal vitamin intakes, known as SONAs

(Suggested Optimal Nutrient Allowances) are often ten times the RDAs (see Figure 2). This is completely consistent with many large-scale supplement studies.

For example, in one trial by Dr Chandra and colleagues, 96 healthy elderly people were given a SONA-level supplement or placebo (dummy pill). Those on supplements had fewer infections, had a stronger immune system on blood tests, and were generally healthier.[9] In another study involving 22,000 pregnant women (some on supplements, some not), those taking supplements had a 75 per cent decrease in birth defects.[10] In a UK study 90 schoolchildren were given either SONA-type supplements, placebos or nothing. Seven months later only those on supplements had 10 per cent raised IQ scores compared to the others.[11]

These are just a few examples of the many studies that show that intakes of nutrients above RDA levels improve the health of infants, children, athletes, pregnant women, the elderly and everyone in between. The library at the Institute for Optimum Nutrition (see Useful Addresses) is full of such research.

	RDA	Suggested Optimal Intake	
	Male/Female	Male/Female 25–50	Male/Female 51+
Vitamin A (retinol)	700/600mcgRE	2000mcgRE	2000mcgRE
Vitamin C	40mg	400mg	800/1000mg
Vitamin E	3/4mcg	400mg	800mg
Vitamin B1 (thiamine)	1/0.8mg	7.5/7.1mg	9.2/9.0mg
Vitamin B2 (riboflavin)	1.3/1.1mg	2.5/2mg	2.5/2mcg
Vitamin B3 (niacin)	17/13mg	30/25mg	30/25mg
Vitamin B6 (pyridoxine)	1.4/1.2mg	10mg	25/20mg
Vitamin B12	1.5µg	2µg	3/2µg
Folic Acid	200µg	800µg	1000µg

(RDAs are Reference Nutrient Intakes from Department of Health, 1991)

Figure 2 – RDAs vs SONAs

In my opinion the weight of current scientific research already shows that an intake of vitamins above RDA levels enhances resistance to infection, improves intellectual performance, and reduces the risk of birth defects, as well as certain cancers and cardiovascular disease. This view is shared by Dr Godfrey Oakley from the US Center for Disease Control and Prevention, who states in an editorial in the *New England Journal of Medicine* entitled 'Eat Right and Take a Multivitamin' that 'the current evidence suggests that people who take [such] supplements and their children are healthier'.[12]

So, how do we achieve these levels? From food? Consider the following: the SONA for vitamin C is 400mg a day. An orange may provide between 0mg and 180mg, the average being around 60mg. Yes, it's true. Some supermarket oranges have spent so long in transit that they contain no vitamin C! The SONA for vitamin E is 400iu. A 100g serving of wheatgerm (about three cups) provides anywhere between 3.2iu and 21iu. The SONA for vitamin A is 3300iu. A large (100g) carrot can provide from 70 to 18,500iu.[13] Even if you ate ten oranges, ten cups of wheatgerm and ten carrots a day you couldn't guarantee achieving these intakes. Why?

◆ THE FOOD SCANDAL

Firstly, food isn't what it used to be. Fruit and vegetables are only as good as the soil they are grown in. Comparative analyses of foods show a marked decrease in mineral levels in food grown in 1991, compared to food grown in 1939. Modern farming robs the soil of nutrients, and doesn't replace them. Food manufacturers are the greatest vitamin robbers. Refining flour, rice and sugar removes more than 77 per cent of its zinc, chromium and manganese (see Figure 3).[14]

	WHITE FLOUR	SUGAR REFINING	RICE POLISHING
Chromium	98%	95%	92%
Zinc	78%	88%	54%
Manganese	86%	89%	75%

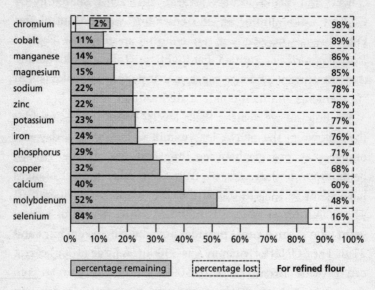

mineral	percentage remaining	percentage lost
chromium	2%	98%
cobalt	11%	89%
manganese	14%	86%
magnesium	15%	85%
sodium	22%	78%
zinc	22%	78%
potassium	23%	77%
iron	24%	76%
phosphorus	29%	71%
copper	32%	68%
calcium	40%	60%
molybdenum	52%	48%
selenium	84%	16%

percentage remaining   percentage lost   For refined flour

Figure 3 – Minerals lost by refining

Fresh, organic food generally has 50–100 per cent higher nutrient levels, as do wholefoods. However, any dried whole-foods, such as beans, lentils and brown rice, will have lost most of their B vitamins for the simple reason that many vita-mins do not survive drying and storing. Then there's cooking. Cooking vegetables results in 20–70 per cent losses in B vitamins.[15] Generally, frying, which involves the highest temperatures, is most destructive to the fat-soluble vitamins A, C and E. Boiling foods will cause a gradual loss in water-soluble B vitamins and vitamin C as well as minerals – which all leach into the water. The temperature will also destroy some of these nutrients over time, so low heat for as short a time as possible is the least destructive method of cooking. For very fibrous vegetables there may even be advantages to light cooking (such as steaming) because this can liberate nutrients.

The ideal diet seems to be closest to the diet we ate during most of our evolution, namely raw, fresh organic fruit, vegetables, nuts and seeds, with fresh organic meat, fish or eggs.

◆ NUTRITION AND EVOLUTION

According to Professor Michael Crawford, co-author of *Nutrition and Evolution – The Driving Force*, the environment in which a species develops is a major factor determining its evolution.[16] Growing evidence suggests that, during a critical period in our ancestors' evolution, we exploited the nutrient-rich environment of the water's edge, eating mussels, shellfish and fish. This diet provided the high levels of essential fats and nutrients needed to develop our extraordinarily complex brain and nervous system. In other words, we picked the best spot as far as nutrition was concerned.

The better our intake of essential nutrients, the greater chance we have, as individuals, of achieving our full potential, and, as a species, of evolving, rather than 'devolving'. One way of guaranteeing an optimal intake of nutrients is to supplement a wholefood diet with beneficial amounts of nutrients which are almost impossible to get from today's food alone.

◆ TO C OR NOT TO C

One 'devolution' which may have occurred, according to Nobel prizewinner Dr Linus Pauling, is the inability of primates to produce vitamin C. All other animals (with a few exceptions) make massive amounts of vitamin C from sugar. The amount they produce is equivalent to between 3000 and 16,000mg per day. That's a little different from the RDA of 60mg and more consistent with the levels known to enhance immune function and minimise the risk of cancer.[17] In fact, vitamin C producing animals are completely immune to some types of cancer and viral diseases. Dr Pauling believes that we used to make vitamin C like other animals, but, when eating a fruit-rich diet, lost the ability because we could eat enough. Now that we no longer live in a tropical jungle, most of us are deficient, as shown by the high incidence of infections and diseases such as cancer which are associated with poor-functioning immune systems.[18] While a gorilla can eat 3000mg a day (66 oranges), it is easier for us to take three 1000mg vitamin C tablets.

◆ THE POLLUTION FACTOR

One particular aspect of modern life makes the 'well-balanced diet' approach obsolete – our unavoidable intake of a vast cocktail of 'anti-nutrients'. More than ten million man-made chemicals have been invented in the last century. In the last 50 years, 3500 more have been added to our food supply.[19] These increase our need for nutrients. For example, the food colouring tartrazine is an antagonist of zinc.[20] So too is unavoidable lead pollution, principally from exhaust fall-out, and cadmium, principally from cigarettes. Modern man has 1000 times the lead level of our jungle-dwelling ancestors.[21]

Other unavoidable 'anti-nutrients' include free radicals from normal body processes, as well as industrial and car pollution. These use up antioxidant nutrients (see Chapter 6) at an alarming rate. To a certain extent, one can limit one's intake of anti-nutrients by avoiding foods with chemical additives, not smoking and staying away from pollution, but there is no such thing as total protection from anti-nutrients. We are living in a very different world from that of our ancestors.

Since all species evolve depending on their access to nutrients, the greater the intake of nutrients the human race receives the better it will adapt and evolve. The evidence – shown by increasing worldwide disease rates – is that we are neither adapting fast enough to the increasing levels of anti-nutrients in our environment, nor adapting our environment (including our diet) to our current needs. Adding vitamin and mineral supplements to a 'well-balanced', unrefined diet is intelligent 'adaptation' and the only sure way to guarantee optimal, or even RDA, intakes of nutrients.

◆ HOW MUCH IS ENOUGH?

ACE PROTECTION

The optimal intake of vitamin A is likely to be at least double the RDA. Even higher levels of beta-carotene (the precursor of vitamin A found in vegetables) may confer extra benefit. The optimal level of vitamin C (rich in fruit) and E (rich in seeds and nuts) is at least ten times the RDA. A 1000mg tablet of vitamin C, the level recommended for a post-menopausal woman, is equivalent to 22 oranges, making supplementation essential. These important antioxidant vitamins, A, C and E, reduce our risk of cancer, heart disease and premature ageing (see Chapter 6 for more on this).

B VITAL

For many of the eight essential B vitamins, optimal levels are again around ten times the RDAs. B vitamins are needed to make energy in every single cell of the body. Even short-term deficiency can result in a decline in mental and physical energy. The best food sources are again fruits and vegetables. However, the only guaranteed way to meet optimal nutritional needs is to take a daily multivitamin and mineral supplement. RDAs, it seems, are only recommended for those who want to stay in average poor health (see Chapter 5 for more on this).

ELEMENTAL HEALTH

The most commonly deficient minerals are magnesium, iron, zinc and chromium. All these are found in wholefoods and they are all seriously reduced when foods are highly processed. Each day, we need at least 350mg of magnesium, found in nuts, seeds, crunchy and leafy vegetables. Iron and zinc are both found in seeds, as well as meat. Chromium, for which no RDA has yet been established, helps the body derive energy from glucose. The more sugar you eat, the more chromium you use up. So chromium levels improve by eating wholefoods and avoiding sugar (see Chapter 3 for more on this).

◆ HOW MUCH DO YOU NEED?

If you want to realise your full potential, mentally and physically, it is essential to find out your optimum nutritional requirements. Since 1980, the Institute for Optimum Nutrition has been developing and refining a precise system for analysing people's individual nutrient needs. This system is now used by qualified nutritionists all over the world and more than 30,000 people have benefited from it.

What follows is a simplified version of this system, based on symptoms of deficiency. It provides a useful assessment of what you need for optimum health and is a good starting point. It is not, however, the same as having a personal assessment of your nutritional needs by a clinical nutritionist. This is definitely preferable, and essential for anyone who is currently unwell or suffering from a diagnosed disease. A directory of clinical nutritionists, qualified to assess your individual needs for optimum health, is available from ION (see page 180).

At least eight factors affect your optimum nutritional requirements. Those such as age, sex and the amount of exercise you do are easy to assess. But the effects of pollution, your past health history and, of course, the nutrients (and anti-nutrients) supplied in your diet are not so straightforward to work out. But all these factors and more must be taken into account. Essentially, there are four possible methods of assessment: analyse your diet; run biochemical tests; look at your lifestyle; and analyse symptoms of deficiency.

Deficiency means a lack of efficiency (i.e. less than 100 per cent health). Deficiency symptom analysis is the most under-estimated method of working out nutritional needs. It is based on over 200 signs and symptoms that have been found in cases of slight vitamin or mineral deficiency. For example, mouth ulcers are associated with vitamin A deficiency, and muscle cramps with magnesium deficiency. Symptoms such as these can be early warning signs, showing us that our bodies are not working perfectly. However, while deficiencies in vitamins C, B3 or B5 would all result in fatigue because they are involved in the production of energy, being low in energy doesn't necessarily mean you're deficient in these vitamins – perhaps you are just working too hard or sleeping badly. However, if you have five different symptoms, all associated with B3 deficiency, then it is much more likely that you need more vitamin B3 to reach optimum health. Check your own status using our special questionnaire.

◆ HOW WELL-NOURISHED ARE YOU?

CHECK YOUR VITAMIN STATUS

Underline each symptom that you often experience. An <u>underlined</u> symptom scores one point. A **<u>bold underlined</u>** symptom scores two points. Write your score for each nutrient in the box. A score of five or more means your needs are higher than the suggested optimal nutrient allowances. Many symptoms occur more than once. This is because they can be the result of many nutrient deficiencies.

VITAMIN PROFILE

Vitamin A
- **Mouth ulcers**
- Poor night vision
- Acne
- **Frequent colds or infections**
- Dry flaky skin
- Dandruff
- Thrush or cystitis
- Diarrhoea   *Your score* ☐

Vitamin D
- **Arthritis or osteoporosis**
- Backache
- Tooth decay
- Hair loss
- **Muscle twitching or spasms**
- **Joint pain or stiffness**
- Weak bones   *Your score* ☐

Vitamin E
- Lack of sex drive
- **Exhaustion after light exercise**
- **Easy bruising**
- Slow wound healing
- Varicose veins
- Poor skin elasticity
- Loss of muscle tone
- Infertility   *Your score* ☐

Vitamin C
- **Frequent colds**
- Lack of energy
- **Frequent infections**
- Bleeding or tender gums
- Easy bruising
- Nose bleeds
- Slow wound healing
- Red pimples on skin   *Your score* ☐

Questionnaire continues

Vitamin B1 (Thiamin)
- Tender muscles
- Eye pains
- Irritability
- Poor concentration
- 'Prickly' legs
- Poor memory
- Stomach pains
- Constipation
- Tingling hands
- Rapid heartbeat   *Your score* ☐

Vitamin B2 (Riboflavin)
- **Bloodshot, burning or gritty eyes**
- **Sensitivity to bright lights**
- Sore tongue
- Cataracts
- Dull or oily hair
- Eczema or dermatitis
- Split nails
- Cracked lips   *Your score* ☐

Vitamin B3 (Niacin)
- Lack of energy
- Diarrhoea
- Insomnia
- Headaches or migraines
- Poor memory

- Anxiety or tension
- Depression
- Irritability
- Bleeding or tender gums
- Acne   *Your score* ☐

Vitamin B5 (Pantothenic acid)
- Muscle tremors, cramps or spasms
- Apathy
- Poor concentration
- **Burning feet or tender heels**
- Nausea or vomiting
- Lack of energy
- Exhaustion after light exercise
- Anxiety or tension
- Teeth grinding   *Your score* ☐

Vitamin B6 (Pyridoxine)
- **Infrequent dream recall**
- **Water retention**
- Tingling hands
- Depression or nervousness
- Irritability
- Muscle tremors, cramps or spasms
- **Lack of energy**   *Your score* ☐

Questionnaire continues

Vitamin B12

- Poor hair condition
- Eczema or dermatitis
- Mouth over-sensitive to hot or cold
- Irritability
- Anxiety or tension
- **Lack of energy**
- Constipation
- Tender or sore muscles
- Pale skin   *Your score* ☐

Folic acid

- Eczema
- Cracked lips
- Prematurely greying hair
- Anxiety or tension
- Poor memory
- **Lack of energy**
- Depression
- Poor appetite
- Stomach pains   *Your score* ☐

Biotin

- **Dermatitis or dry skin**
- **Poor hair condition**
- **Prematurely greying hair**
- **Tender or sore muscles**
- **Poor appetite or nausea** *Your score* ☐

MINERAL PROFILE

Calcium
- Muscle cramps, tremors or spasms
- Insomnia or nervousness
- Joint pain or arthritis
- Tooth decay
- High blood pressure   *Your score* ☐

Magnesium
- Muscle cramps, tremors or spasms
- Muscles weakness
- Insomnia, nervousness or hyperactivity
- High blood pressure
- Irregular or rapid heartbeat
- Constipation
- Fits or convulsions
- Breast tenderness or water retention
- Depression or confusion   *Your score* ☐

Iron
- Pale skin
- Sore tongue
- Fatigue or listlessness
- Loss of appetite or nausea
- Heavy periods or blood loss   *Your score* ☐

Questionnaire continues

Zinc
- Decline in sense of taste or smell
- White marks on more than two fingernails
- Frequent infections
- Stretch marks
- Acne or greasy skin   *Your score* ☐

Manganese
- Muscle twitches
- Childhood 'growing pains'
- Dizziness or poor sense of balance
- Fits or convulsions
- Sore knees   *Your score* ☐

Selenium
- Family history of cancer
- Signs of premature ageing
- Cataracts
- High blood pressure
- Frequent infections   *Your score* ☐

Chromium
- Excessive or cold sweats
- Dizziness/irritability after six hours without food
- Need for frequent meals
- Cold hands
- Need for excessive sleep/drowsiness during the day

    Your score ☐

Now use your scores to work out the ideal daily level to supplement for each nutrient, using the chart opposite.

YOUR TOTAL SCORE		SCORE				WHAT YOU NEED
		0–4	5–6	7–8	9 or more	
	A	7500	10000	15000	20000	ius
	D	200	400	600	800	ius
	E	100	300	500	1000	ius
	C	1000	2000	3000	4000	mg
	B1	25	50	75	100	mg
	B2	25	50	75	100	mg
	B3	50	75	100	150	mg
	B5	50	100	200	300	mg
	B6	50	100	200	250	mg
	B12	5	10	50	100	mcg
	F A	50	100	200	400	mcg
	Biotin	50	100	150	200	mcg
	GLAΩ6	–	150	225	300	mg
	EPA/Ω3	–	800	1600	2400	mg
	Cal	150	300	450	600	mg
	Mag	75	150	225	300	mg
	Iron	10	15	20	25	mg
	Zinc	10	15	20	25	mg
	Man	2.5	5	10	15	mg
	Sel	25	50	75	100	mcg
	Chro	20	50	100	200	mcg

◆ YOUR PERSONAL SUPPLEMENT PROGRAMME

Once you've worked out your score, you can use the table to calculate the ideal level for you to supplement. These levels already take into account roughly the amount you're likely to get from food, so the figures relate not to your ideal daily intake but to actual supplementation. In case you are wondering, you don't have to take 30 different supplements every day! Your needs can be compressed into four or five different tablets or capsules, each combining the above nutrients. The most common combinations are a multivitamin (containing vitamins A, B, C, D and E), and a multimineral for all the minerals. Vitamin C is usually taken separately, since the basic optimum requirement of 1000mg (1g) makes quite a large tablet without adding any more nutrients. I also take an antioxidant nutrient (see Chapter 6). Choosing the right formula is an art in itself, explained in Part 3.

◆ WHAT ABOUT CHILDREN?

Supplements are equally important for children, although they require different amounts. The best way to optimally nourish an infant is to optimally nourish the breast-feeding mother. Once breast-feeding stops (with the arrival of teeth and an increasing appetite), you can introduce chewable vitamin and mineral supplements. A rough guide to the levels you should be looking for in a children's chewable supplement are shown opposite (Figure 4). You should also check that the supplement is free from colourings and sugar. Once a child turns 11, you can give two-thirds of the adult dosage, calculated using the system in this book. From age 14 use the adult dose, but note that the system bumps up nutrient requirements for vitamins A, D, B6, biotin, calcium and zinc between the ages of 14 to 16.

Vitamins	Less than 1	Age 1	2	3–4	5–6	7–8	9–11	12–13	
A (retinol and beta-carotene)	2500	2800	3200	3600	4000	4400	4800	5500	ius
(in mcgRE)	750	840	970	1080	1200	1320	1440	1650	mcg
D	200	200	200	200	200	200	200	300	ius
E	10	15	20	30	40	50	60	70	ius
C	100	175	250	325	400	475	550	625	mg
B1 (thiamine)	3	4	5	6	8	12	16	20	mg
B2 (riboflavin)	3	4	5	6	8	12	16	20	mg
B3 (niacin)	7	8	9	10	15	20	25	35	mg
B5 (pantothenic acid)	7	8	9	10	15	20	25	35	mg
B6 (pyridoxine)	7	8	9	10	15	20	25	35	mg
B12	3	4	5	6	7	8	9	10	mcg
Folic acid	50	55	60	65	70	80	90	100	mcg
Biotin	20	25	30	35	40	45	50	55	mcg
Minerals									
Calcium	150	150	150	150	150	150	150	150	mg
Magnesium	25	35	45	55	65	75	85	95	mg
Iron	2	2	3	4	5	6	7	8	mg
Zinc	3	4	5	6	7	8	10	12	mg
Manganese	0.7	1	1.3	1.5	1.7	1.8	1.9	2	mg
Chromium	10	12.5	15	17.5	20	22.5	25	30	mcg
Selenium	7	8	10	12	14	16	18	20	mcg

Reproduced with the kind permission of Natural Justice

Figure 4 – Optimum Nutrient Amounts to Supplement from the Age of One to Thirteen

part 2

chapter 2

ABC of Vitamins

First, there was carbohydrate, fat and protein; then there were vitamins. One by one, the food factors that prevent disease have been isolated and called 'vitamins': vitamin A for preventing blindness, vitamin C for preventing scurvy, and so on. The erroneous popular belief is that we only need enough of each nutrient to prevent these severe deficiency diseases. In truth, each vitamin has many roles to play in maintaining our health and each works in combination with others. For this reason the basis of any supplement programme is a good high-strength multivitamin and multi-mineral. This chapter explores the key role of each vitamin and what you should expect to find in your multivitamin.

◆ VITAMIN A

Vitamin A is vital for healthy immunity, is important in all growth and repair, and acts as a potent antioxidant (for more on antioxidants see Chapter 6).

Vitamin A is essential for the growth and maintenance of

skin (inside and out), the lungs, gastro-intestinal tract, womb, and so on. It is known as the growth vitamin, because it is necessary for the production of growth hormone, which in turn is responsible, not only for growth, but for maintaining an active thymus gland which is a critical part of the body's immune system.

Vitamin A is a powerful anti-viral vitamin, mainly because its inclusion in cell walls makes them stronger and more resistant to viral attack. It is particularly important for areas with a high risk of infection, such as the respiratory system, the gut and the genito-urinary tract. Body secretions, like sweat, tears and saliva, as well as the immune system's cells, all need vitamin A for the production of lysozyme, a protective antibacterial enzyme. Vitamin A is helpful in cancer prevention and treatment of pre-cancerous conditions. For example, people with lung cancer have been found to have much lower than normal vitamin A and beta-carotene levels in their blood. People who regularly suffer from conjunctivitis are probably deficient in vitamin A (as well as vitamin C). You need more when you are fighting an infection (especially viral), if you smoke, if you are exposed to pollution, or if you are under considerable stress. This vitamin also helps heal many skin conditions, from acne to eczema.

The first signs of vitamin A deficiency are skin complaints such as dry, flaky skin, dandruff and acne. Frequent infections, cystitis or diarrhoea are other indications. Other symptoms include frequent mouth ulcers and poor night vision. In more pronounced vitamin A deficiency children's growth rate slows down and eyes become dry and irritated. In severe deficiency, cataracts develop (eventually leading to blindness).

Good food sources of vitamin A (or its precursor beta-carotene) are liver, carrots, watercress, sweet potatoes, melon, pumpkin, mangoes and other red/orange foods.

In supplements, vitamin A comes in two forms: retinol or beta-carotene. Retinol is found in animal sources, although it can be artificially made. Retinyl palmitate, from palm oil, is a vegetarian version of this vitamin. Retinol is a direct source of vitamin A and is stored in the liver, so supplementing retinol is the quickest way to increase body stores. This has the potential disadvantage, however, of leading to excessive liver stores and toxicity (see Chapter 14).

When supplements of vitamin A are needed, they are best taken in the form of beta-carotene, as this form is not toxic and is only made into vitamin A as the body requires it. On average, you need six times as much beta-carotene to make 1 unit of retinol.

Vitamin A measurements are a little tricky. This is because beta-carotene is not actually vitamin A, but can be turned into vitamin A by the body. So, to indicate the equivalent effect of a certain amount of beta-carotene, as compared to vitamin A (retinol), we use a unit called a 'µgRE'. This stands for 'micrograms of Retinol Equivalent', meaning that this amount of beta-carotene has the equivalent effect of Xµg of retinol. In fact, 6mcg of beta-carotene is equivalent in potency to 1mcg of retinol and is therefore written as 1mcgRE of beta-carotene. If a supplement contains both vitamin A and beta-carotene, add together the two amounts of 'µgRE' to work out the total vitamin A dose provided.

Beta-carotene is also an antioxidant in its own right, as is retinol, so supplementing beta-carotene effectively gives you two different kinds of antioxidants. Diabetics are better off supplementing vitamin A or cod liver oil (which is a concentrated source of vitamin A), as they cannot convert beta-carotene into vitamin A. Supplements need to be taken with vitamin E to be most effective, as vitamins A and E protect each other.

Optimal Intake: 7400μgRE
From Diet: 820μgRE   **From Supplements:** 2500–6600μgRE

◆ VITAMIN B

The main role of the B vitamins is to help turn the food you eat into energy (for more on the B vitamins see Chapter 5). Vitamin B complex is a family of eight essential nutrients. These are used by just about all our cells for a great many of the body's chemical reactions. Deficiency symptoms are therefore very varied, although the first signs are always mental and emotional (such as depression, anxiety, moodiness and difficulty concentrating), probably because the brain is absolutely dependent on getting a 24-hour supply of these vitamins. Energy is often low too, because B vitamins are needed to make it from the food we eat. A host of other symptoms may also appear, like headaches, pre-menstrual tension, bad breath, dandruff, eczema, water retention, weight problems and sensitivity to light.

Vitamin B1 (thiamin) is especially important for digestion and the body's use of carbohydrate and sugar. High sugar consumers are frequently deficient in B1. People who exercise a lot need more vitamin B2 (riboflavin) which helps control the acidity generated when muscles work hard. Vitamin B3 (niacin) has the remarkable ability to help remove unwanted cholesterol and is vasodilatory (i.e. dilates blood vessels, causing blushing) at high doses. Deficiency leads to mental health problems. B3 also helps alleviate headaches and arthritis.

Vitamin B5 (pantothenic acid) is needed to make stress hormones and can help those with high stress levels or concentration problems (see Chapter 8). Vitamin B6 (pyridoxine) is essential for all protein use in the body and has been helpful in a variety of conditions, from PMS to carpal tunnel syndrome (a strain condition affecting nerves in the wrist) and cardiovascular disease.

Folic acid is now recognised as essential for the prevention of neural tube defects in pregnancy and the UK government recommends that pregnant women supplement 400mcg. Optimal levels, especially in the elderly, may be much higher. However, bear in mind that folic acid supplementation can mask B12 deficiency anaemia. So it's best to supplement extra folic acid with vitamin B12. During pregnancy folic acid is also necessary for all cell division, and therefore important for healing after the birth.

Vitamins B6, B12 and folic acid are all vital for utilising protein, and thus for general repair and maintenance. Deficiency in any of these nutrients leads to blood abnormalities and anaemia. These three, plus pantothenic acid (B5), boost the immune system and are necessary for antibody production, helping immune cells to work efficiently. Since bacteria in the digestive tract make some B vitamins, you will need to take in more after a course of antibiotics, which kills off many of these 'good' bacteria. Anyone who is highly stressed, or who has a lot of sugar, alcohol or refined food, robs themselves of B vitamins.

Probably one of the most reliable physical guides to severe B vitamin deficiency is the mouth, and in particular the tongue (change in size, deep fissures, very smooth and sore, coating or off-colour). You may also get cracked, sore lips and mouth corners. The obvious deficiency in the mouth will be extended to other areas of digestion, showing up as excessive gas and indigestion.

Good food sources of B vitamins are most vegetables (especially watercress, mushrooms and cabbage), legumes (such as lentils and alfalfa sprouts), fish and chicken. Vitamin B12 is only found in 'animal' products, including oysters, fish, poultry and dairy produce.

When supplementing B vitamins it is best either to make sure you have good levels of each in a multivitamin or to take a B complex, which gives a good balance of them all. Sometimes a single B vitamin needs to be supplemented for a short time to restore a balance, but it should be taken with a B complex or multivitamin. A good B complex supplement provides somewhere between 25 and 75mg of B1, B2, B3, B5 and B6, plus 10µg of B12, 100µg of biotin and 100–400µg of folic acid. Under most circumstances you can get enough B vitamins in a high-strength multivitamin.

B1 Optimal Intake: 50mg
From Diet: 1.26mg   **From Supplements:** 25–50mg

B2 Optimal Intake: 50mg
From Diet: 1.6mg   **From Supplements:** 25–50mg

B3 Optimal Intake: 75mg
From Diet: 25.5mg   **From Supplements:** 25–50mg

B5 Optimal Intake: 100mg
From Diet: 4–10mg   **From Supplements:** 25–100mg

B6 Optimal Intake: 100mg
From Diet: 2mg   **From Supplements:** 50–100mg

B12 Optimal Intake: 20µg
From Diet: 4.9µg   **From Supplements:** 5–20µg

Folic acid Optimal Intake: 500µg

From Diet: 190µg   **From Supplements:** 100–400µg

Biotin Optimal Intake: 150µg

From Diet: 28–100µg   **From Supplements:** 50–100µg

1 VITAMIN C

This is one piece of the jigsaw that will make up your personal supplement programme (see page 138)

Vitamin C is important in energy production; it is a potent antioxidant; it is also essential for collagen and bone formation and is a powerful immune booster (for more on immunity see Chapter 7).

Most animals are able to make vitamin C in the body from glucose. Only humans, other primates, guinea pigs, the Indian fruit-eating bat, and the red-vented bulbul bird do not. All these rely on vitamin C in their diet and would die of scurvy without it.

Humans, and other primates, used to make ascorbic acid in sufficient quantities but lost this ability in the course of evolution; the mutation did not at first pose a great threat, because we had plenty of vitamin C in our diet. But storage and processing now deplete our food of vitamin C, and we eat less fresh fruit than our ancestors did.

Other animals, like gorillas, living in the wild, consume about 4500mg of vitamin C daily in fresh food – 100 times more than the average daily intake for man. Other mammals too, instinctively saturate their blood and tissue with vitamin C and step up their production when they are ill, fighting an infection or under stress. It is possible that infectious diseases, cardiovascular disorders, collagen diseases, cancer and premature ageing are among the many ills which could be prevented if we still had the ability to regulate our vitamin C levels internally.

Good food sources of vitamin C are peppers, broccoli, kiwi fruit, watercress, strawberries, tomatoes and lemons.

Symptoms of vitamin C deficiency include frequent colds and infections, bleeding or receding gums, nose bleeds, red pimples on the skin, easy bruising, slow wound healing, and lack of energy. If you have some of these symptoms you are well advised to up your intake of this vital vitamin.

Whilst many studies confirm the benefits of supplementing vitamin C, others do not, probably due to dosage differences. A useful indication of vitamin C requirements is 'bowel tolerance'. A healthy adult will tolerate up to 4000mg of vitamin C before getting diarrhoea. During a bout of flu, this tolerance may go up to 8000mg, while for a person with cancer or AIDS, it could be 20,000–30,000mg a day.

Age is another major factor. Our absorption of vitamin C declines considerably with age, though in old animals production is not much different from their young. Older people need more vitamin C spread out in small amounts over the day. It's worth supplementing more vitamin C during winter when need is higher and dietary supply, in terms of fresh fruit, tends to be less. Those who both smoke and drink alcohol need much more vitamin C. Smokers on average have 25 per cent less vitamin C in the blood than similar non-smokers on the same diet. Heavy drinkers also need extra vitamin C and zinc, as both are necessary for the production of alcohol dehydrogenase, the liver enzyme which detoxifies alcohol. Aspirin also depletes the body's vitamin C reserves.

A 1000mg dose of vitamin C is equivalent to 22 oranges – in other words supplementation is essential, as you would be hard pressed to eat enough food to get that much. The RDA for vitamin C is 60mg – the equivalent of an orange a day (assuming the orange really does contain that much, and many don't). Supplements are best taken with bioflavonoids, which help to strengthen the effect of vitamin C – fresh fruit and vegetables contain both.

An ideal daily intake of vitamin C is 500–3000mg. It comes in two forms: ascorbic acid and ascorbate. Some people do not tolerate large amounts of ascorbic acid, which is a weak acid. Most people prefer the more alkaline form of vitamin C, known as ascorbate (e.g. calcium ascorbate or magnesium ascorbate). The only problem with taking large amounts of ascorbate is that it can tend to neutralise stomach acid, which interferes with protein digestion. So, if you are supplementing several grams of ascorbate (for instance to fight a cold), don't take it at mealtimes.

Optimal Intake: 1000 to 3000mg
From Diet: 52mg   **From Supplements:** 1000–3000mg

◆ VITAMIN D

When the sun's ultraviolet light (UV) hits the skin, it changes the form of cholesterol in the skin into cholecalciferol, which is the natural form of vitamin D (known as D3) also found in fish oil. Other forms are synthetic versions.

Our skin colour determines the amount of UV light we let through and the amount of vitamin D made. Black skin only allows 3–36 per cent of the UV through, and white skin 52–72 per cent. In general, we make less vitamin D in winter because we have less exposure to sunlight. Supplementing fish oil is therefore particularly good for children and the elderly, because they need vitamin D for bone growth and repair (as well as calcium and magnesium). Many degenerative bone problems could be avoided with the right diet, exercise and exposure to sunshine.

Good food sources of vitamin D are herring, mackerel, salmon, cheese and other dairy produce. Natural supplements, like fish oil, are the best food sources. Vitamin D is fat-soluble and so is stored in the body. It is possible to take too much, so sunlight and fish should be used wherever possible and it should only be supplemented when really necessary, although it is a good idea to take a multivitamin that includes some.

Optimal Intake: 20µg
From Diet: 5µg   **From Supplements:** 5–20µg

♦ VITAMIN E

This is one of the most essential antioxidants (see Chapter 6), as it helps the body to use oxygen properly.

Unfortunately, these days we are so obsessed with increasing the shelf-life of foods that we seem to want them to last longer than the people who eat them! Vitamin E is an essential nutrient, but it is often removed if the food is to be kept for a long time. (Although it is a natural antioxidant, it goes off faster than the artificial ones which are used to replace it.)

Vitamin E is necessary for a normal immunity and antibody response. As an antioxidant in our fat layers, it neutralises free radicals and works with other nutrients to improve our resistance to infection. It is very effective in protecting us from air pollution, particularly that due to exhausts, air purifiers or deodorisers which generate ozone.

There are many reasons to supplement vitamin E. It reduces the risk of cancer and heart disease and slows down the ageing process, as well as boosting immunity. These benefits are rarely seen below 100mg (150iu) a day. Above 400mg (600iu) there seems little extra benefit to be derived from vitamin E.

The first signs of vitamin E deficiency are circulatory – easy bruising, slow wound healing, varicose veins. Loss of muscle tone and poor skin elasticity are also associated with deficiency, as are infertility and lack of sex drive.

Good food sources of vitamin E are unrefined corn oil, sunflower seeds, sesame seeds, wheatgerm, tuna, beans and peas.

Optimal Intake: 660mg
From Diet: 5mg   **From Supplements:** 66–660mg

◆ VITAMIN K

Vitamin K is often excluded from supplements because it is normally made in sufficient amounts by bacteria in the digestive tract. It is essential for normal blood clotting. At birth, infants are given vitamin K on the grounds that they have yet to establish intestinal bacteria and, if the mother's own bacteria is disrupted (for example, after a course of antibiotics) and her diet is deficient of food sources, her breast milk could be deficient too. As a consequence, such infants can bleed at birth and be unable to stop bleeding due to the lack of this essential clotting factor.

Good food sources of vitamin K are cauliflower, Brussels sprouts, beans, peas and broccoli.

2 MULTIVITAMIN SUPPLEMENTS

This is one piece of the jigsaw that will make up your personal supplement programme (see page 138)

A good daily multivitamin supplement should provide roughly the following amounts of each vitamin. With some brands, you'll need to take two or three actual pills to achieve these levels.

A (retinol/beta-carotene)	2500 – 6600µgRE (7500–20,000iu)
D	5 – 20µg (200–800iu)
E	66 – 660mg (100 –1000iu)
C	100 – 300mg
B1 (thiamin)	25 – 50mg
B2 (riboflavin)	25 – 50mg
B3 (niacin)	25 – 50mg
B5 (pantothenic acid)	25 – 100mg
B6 (pyridoxine)	50 – 100mg
Folic acid	100 – 400µg
B12 (cyanocobalamin)	5 – 20µg
Biotin	50 – 100µg

chapter 3

Minerals,
from Calcium to Zinc

ore than a hundred years ago a Russian chemist called Mendeleyev noticed that all the basic constituents of matter – the elements – could be arranged in a pattern according to their chemical properties. From this he produced the Periodic Table. There are many gaps where elements should be, but over the years these missing elements have been discovered. All matter, including the human body, is made out of these elements.

Some of them are gases (like oxygen and hydrogen), some are liquids and some are solids (such as iron, zinc and chromium). A total of 96 per cent of your body is made up of carbon, hydrogen, oxygen and nitrogen (which form carbohydrate, protein and fat) and vitamins. The remaining 4 per cent is made from minerals.

Most minerals help to regulate and balance our body chemistry. Calcium, phosphorus and magnesium (which are the major constituents of bone) and sodium and potassium (which control the water balance in your body) are called 'macrominerals' because we need relatively large amounts each day

(300–3000mg). The remaining elements are called 'trace minerals' because we need only traces (30mcg–30mg). These minerals are required in tiny amounts compared to carbon, hydrogen and oxygen. For instance, a 63kg man needs 400g of carbohydrate a day and only 40mcg of chromium (a millionth of the amount). Yet chromium is no less important to his physical well-being.

◆ MINERAL DEFICIENCY IS WIDESPREAD

Minerals are originally extracted from the soil by plants. Like vitamins, we can obtain them directly from plants or indirectly via meat; and, like vitamins, they are frequently deficient in our modern diet. There are three primary reasons for this:

1. MINERAL LEVELS IN NATURAL FOODS ARE DECLINING

This is partly because soil gradually loses its mineral content through over-farming, unless the farmer replaces the minerals by using mineral-rich manure. Many of the minerals that pass from plants to us are not actually needed to make the plants grow so there is no profit incentive for the farmer. The minerals that are added in fertiliser (NPK-nitrogen, phosphate, potassium) make the plants grow faster, and, in the case of phosphate, bind to trace minerals like zinc and make them harder for the plants to take up. Analyses of mineral levels in plants in 1939 compared to 1991 show, on average, a drop of 22 per cent. (The accuracy of this data is, however, a little suspect, as analytical methods have improved dramatically in the intervening period.)

2. ESSENTIAL MINERALS ARE REFINED OUT OF FOOD

Refining food to make white rice, white flour and white sugar removes up to 90 per cent of the trace minerals. Why, you might wonder, do we refine foods like flour? To make it unable to support the life of a weevil. That's what we eat when we eat white flour – food that won't support the life of an insect. Refining foods makes them longer-lasting and thus more profitable. There are laws about a few nutrients so that foods like refined cereals must meet a minimum requirement and thus have some calcium, iron and B vitamins put back in. As a selling point, the packet often boasts 'enriched' or 'with added vitamins and minerals' which of course wouldn't be necessary if the food wasn't refined in the first place.

3. OUR MINERAL NEEDS ARE INCREASING

Dr Stephen Davies from London's Biolab Medical Unit has analysed over 65,000 samples of blood, hair and sweat over the past 15 years. Without exception, mineral levels for lead, cadmium, aluminium and mercury increase with age, while the levels of magnesium, zinc, chromium, manganese and selenium decrease. The toxic minerals are 'anti-nutrients' which compete with essential minerals. As we age, the toxic elements accumulate and push out the essential minerals. We need more minerals today to protect us from the unavoidable toxic minerals that surround us due to pollution of food, air and water.

So it is hardly surprising that most of us are deficient in minerals, for the reasons above. Also, many of us choose to eat the wrong foods, such as refined bread, pasta and cereal, and avoid mineral-rich foods such as seeds and nuts. The average dietary intake of zinc (7.5mg) is half the RDA of 15mg. The recommended intake for a breast-feeding woman is 25mg, more than three times the average intake, leaving most breast-fed infants hopelessly deficient in a mineral that is essential for all growth processes including intellectual development.

The average intakes of iron and magnesium are also well below the RDAs; and, although no RDAs exist for manganese, chromium and selenium, dietary intakes are certainly below estimates of what we need for optimal health and are well worth supplementing. Other trace elements, such as iodine, copper, boron, molybdenum and vanadium, should also be supplemented. Calcium is worth 'topping up' because optimal levels may be a little higher than those that can easily be achieved by diet, especially for those who don't have dairy products on a regular basis. The minerals phosphorus, potassium and sodium are easily obtained in sufficient quantities from diet so there is no need to supplement these.

◆ BORON

Boron is an abundant trace element in soil, food and in man. Boron is an essential element for plants, possibly because of its effect on the control of plant growth hormones.

Although it has not yet been proven to be essential in man, boron is found in the human body. It appears to be more concentrated in the thyroid and parathyroid glands which may suggest a role in their function. Animal studies point to an interaction between boron and calcium balance. Deficiency of vitamin D increases the need for boron and it is suspected that boron is somehow involved with the action of the parathyroid hormone, which helps maintain calcium within bone. Animals given boron supplements were found to be much less susceptible to the effects of magnesium deficiency. And, according to Professor Derek Bryce-Smith of the University of Reading, 'It would be surprising if such effects were confined to the animal kingdom.'[1] In plants boron is involved with the transport of calcium. Because of its link with calcium, boron may be beneficial for arthritis sufferers and could help prevent osteoporosis.

These early studies of boron used daily supplements of 3–9mg, given as sodium borate. At much higher levels (above 500mg) boron becomes toxic, as do most minerals. Some supplements now combine calcium, or calcium and magnesium, with boron. It would appear that supplementing up to 3mg a day, together with a high fruit and vegetable diet, would provide a more than optimal intake of this potentially important trace element.

Good food sources of boron are vegetables, apples, pears, tomatoes, soya, prunes, raisins, dates and honey.

Optimal Intake: 4mg
From Diet: 2mg **From Supplements:** 1–3mg

◆ CALCIUM

Nearly 1.4kg of your body weight is calcium and 99 per cent of this is in your bones and teeth. Calcium provides the rigid structure of the skeleton, so it is particularly necessary for children whose bones are growing, and also for the elderly whose ability to absorb calcium gradually declines. The remaining 10 or so grams of calcium are in the nerves, muscles and blood. It is needed, along with magnesium, for nerves and muscles to 'fire'. It also helps the blood to clot and helps maintain the right acid–alkaline balance in the body.

The average diet provides marginally less than the RDA for calcium. Most of this comes from milk and cheese, which are poor sources of magnesium (which is needed to balance calcium use). However, green vegetables (such as kale, spinach, turnip greens, cabbage and parsley), pulses, nuts, seeds, wholegrains and water provide significant quantities of both calcium and magnesium. Our ancestors, before they started rearing animals for milk, relied on these foods for their calcium. Good sources of calcium are foods such as green vegetables, almonds, sesame seeds and pumpkin seeds.

Our ability to use calcium depends not only on how much we take in but also on how well we absorb it. The amount we absorb depends on the food but we normally absorb around 20–30 per cent of the total calcium content. Its balance in the body is improved by adequate vitamin D intake and by weight-bearing exercise. It is made worse by a deficiency of vitamin D, exposure to lead, consumption of alcohol, coffee and tea or a lack of hydrochloric acid in the stomach. The presence of naturally occurring chemicals called phytates (found in grains) and excessive phosphorous or fat in the diet also interferes with absorption. In addition, excessive protein consumption causes loss of calcium from the bones.

Symptoms of calcium deficiency include muscle cramps, tremors or spasms, insomnia, nervousness, joint pain, osteoarthritis, tooth decay and high blood pressure. Severe deficiency causes osteoporosis, or porous bones. However, this is more likely to be connected with hormone imbalances and protein excess, both of which affect calcium utilisation in the body.

Optimal Intake: 800–1000mg
From Diet: 500–800mg   **From Supplements:** 150–500mg

◆ CHROMIUM

Chromium is a vital constituent of the 'glucose tolerance factor', a compound produced in the liver which helps transport glucose from the blood to the cells (for more on this see Chapter 5). Vitamin B3 and the amino acids glycine, glutamic acid and cystine are also required for glucose tolerance factor. Since it works with insulin to help stabilise your blood sugar level, the more uneven your blood sugar level the more chromium you use up. Hence, a sugar and stimulant addict, eating refined foods, is most at risk of deficiency.

The average daily intake is below 50mcg, while an optimal intake (certainly for those with blood sugar balance problems) is around 200mcg. Continued stress or frequent sugar consumption deplete the body of chromium. If you eat a lot of refined foods you are also likely to be deficient in this mineral, since it is found in wholegrains, pulses, nuts and seeds, as well as mushrooms, asparagus, brewer's yeast and oysters. Flour has 98 per cent of its chromium removed in the refining process – another reason to stay away from refined foods. Chromium supplements have been used successfully in the treatment of diabetes and glucose intolerance.

Whether or not you can achieve an optimal intake of chromium from diet alone is debatable. It is therefore wise to take supplements as well as eating wholefoods. The best forms of chromium are either picolinate or polynicotinate.

Optimal Intake: 100µg
From Diet: 45µg   **From Supplements:** 20–100µg

◆ COPPER

Copper is both a nutritional and a toxic element. Deficiency is rare, for the simple reason that most of our water supplies are contaminated with copper from copper pipes. Copper is needed for the formation of the insulating sheath around nerves (myelin) and it is also a constituent of one of the body's superoxide dismutase (SOD) enzymes which acts as an anti-oxidant, helping to disarm free radicals. Copper and zinc are strongly antagonistic and a deficiency in zinc may lead to a greater uptake of copper. Likewise, excessive zinc supplementation can induce copper deficiency. Don't supplement more than 2mg a day and always take 10–15 times more zinc.

In reality, excess is a more common problem than deficiency. If you are on a wholefood diet, there's no need to supplement copper, yet it is often included in multimineral tablets. Taking the birth control pill or HRT also increases copper stores. All these factors make it relatively easy to accumulate too much copper, which is associated with schizophrenia, cardiovascular disease and possibly rheumatoid arthritis (although a deficiency of copper has also been associated with rheumatoid arthritis). Copper is involved in an antioxidant enzyme which plays a role in some inflammatory reactions, which may be why too much or too little can result in greater inflammation in those with rheumatoid arthritis. Copper levels rise during pregnancy and it may play a part in bringing on labour and, in excess, post-natal depression.

Good food sources of copper include nuts, seeds, wholegrains and other wholefoods.

Optimal Intake: 2mg
From Diet: 1.5mg   **From Supplements:** 0.25–0.75g

◆ IODINE

Iodine is essential for the body to make thyroxine, the main thyroid hormone that controls your rate of metabolism. Hence a lack of iodine leads to an underactive thyroid, the symptoms of which include weight gain, sluggish digestion and a lack of motivation. Iodine is found in the sea and is deficient in the soil in large land masses. Iodine deficiency is rare these days because we eat food grown from all over the world and because many brands of table salt are enriched with iodine. The best food source is kelp. Supplementing too much iodine has been reported to aggravate acne.

Optimal Intake: 100µg
From Diet: 65µg   **From Supplements:** 20–45µg

◆ IRON

Iron, as the red pigment, haem, is a vital component of haemoglobin which transports oxygen and carbon dioxide to and from cells. Of the iron within us, 60 per cent is in the form of haem iron. This is the form present in meat, which is much more readily absorbed than the non-haem iron present in non-meat food sources. Non-haem iron occurs in the oxidised or ferric state in food, and it can only be absorbed when it has been reduced to the ferrous state (for example by vitamin C) during digestion.

The symptoms of iron deficiency include pale skin, sore tongue, fatigue or listlessness, loss of appetite and nausea. Anaemia is clinically diagnosed by checking haemoglobin levels in the blood. However, symptoms of anaemia can also be caused by a lack of vitamin B12 or folic acid. Iron deficiency anaemia is more likely to occur in women, especially during pregnancy. Since iron is also an antagonist to zinc, supplements containing more than 30mg of iron (over twice the RDA) should not be given without ensuring adequate zinc status. Although it is often supplemented in doses above 50mg, there is little evidence that this is more effective in raising haemoglobin levels than lower doses.

Too much iron may also lead to increased risk of cardiovascular disease. According to a Finnish study on 1900 men, those with higher iron stores were more than twice as likely to have a heart attack.[2] Jerome Sullivan, a pathologist at the Veterans Affairs Medical Center in South Carolina, found a correlation between blood ferritin levels and cardiovascular risk, and thinks this might explain why menstruating women, who lose iron each month, have a lower risk of cardiovascular disease than men, until after the menopause.[3]

Good food sources of iron include liver, meat, pumpkin seeds, parsley, almonds, raisins, prunes and eggs.

Optimal Intake: 15–20mg
From Diet: 9.5mg   **From Supplements:** 10–25mg

◆ MAGNESIUM

Magnesium works together with calcium both in maintaining bone density and in the functioning of nerves and muscles. The average person's diet is relatively high in calcium but deficient in magnesium, because milk (which is our major source of calcium) is low in magnesium. Both calcium and magnesium are present in nuts and seeds, and all green vegetables.

Magnesium is involved as a co-factor in many enzymes in the body, often working with vitamins B1 and B6. It is also involved in protein synthesis (i.e. the making of all proteins including hormones) which may be why it is beneficial in treating pre-menstrual problems. But its most important role is its balance with calcium in maintaining proper nerve and muscle impulses.

A lack of magnesium is strongly associated with cardiovascular disease – individuals dying from coronary heart disease have abnormally low levels of magnesium in the heart. A lack of magnesium causes muscles to go into spasm, and there is considerable evidence (as discussed in B. Altura's article 'Magnesium in Cardiovascular Biology', published in *Scientific American*, pp 28–36, May/June 1995) that some heart attacks are caused not by obstruction of the coronary arteries but by cramping of the arteries, which cuts off the supply of oxygen to the heart.

Good food sources of magnesium include wheatgerm, almonds, cashew nuts, brewer's yeast, buckwheat and Brazil nuts.

Optimal Intake: 400mg
From Diet: 170–260mg   **From Supplements:** 75–225mg

◆ MANGANESE

Manganese is known to be involved in no less than 20 enzyme systems in the body. One of the most critical is an SOD antioxidant enzyme. In animals, manganese deficiency also results in lowered production of insulin – diabetics frequently have low manganese status, and it is thought to be involved in maintaining blood sugar balance. It is also involved in the formation of mucopolysaccharides, a constituent of cartilage. One of the first signs of deficiency is joint pain.

Furthermore, manganese is required for proper brain function. Deficiency has been associated with schizophrenia, Parkinson's disease and epilepsy.

The best food sources include tropical fruits (such as pineapple), blackberries, beans, raspberries, okra, nuts, seeds and wholegrains. Tea is also a significant source of this mineral. Little more than 5 per cent of the manganese we eat in our food is actually absorbed. Similarly, supplements are poorly absorbed. The best forms of manganese are manganese citrate or manganese amino acid chelate.

Optimal Intake: 5mg
From Diet: 1.9–5mg   **From Supplements:** 2.5–5mg

◆ MOLYBDENUM

Molybdenum helps rid the body of free radicals, petrochemicals and sulphites, so it is useful for city-dwellers wanting protection from pollution and car exhaust. Molybdenum-dependent enzymes in the liver are vital to the body's detoxifying ability, so ensuring adequate molybdenum helps your body function optimally.

Good food sources of molybdenum include tomatoes, wheatgerm, pork, lamb, lentils and beans.

Optimal Intake: 100µg
From Diet: 50mcg   **From Supplements:** 20–100µg

◆ SELENIUM

Selenium deficiency was first discovered as the cause of 'Keshan disease' in China. This was a type of heart disease which was prevalent in areas in which the soil was deficient in selenium. It has since been associated with another regional disease, this time in Russia, involving joint degeneration. Perhaps the most significant finding in relation to selenium is its association with a low risk of certain kinds of cancer.

Selenium is the vital constituent of the antioxidant enzyme, glutathione peroxidase. A ten-fold increase in dietary selenium causes a doubling of this enzyme in the body, showing its dependence on this important mineral. Since many oxides are cancer-producing and since cancer cells destroy other cells by releasing oxides, it is probably selenium's role in glutathione peroxidase that gives it its protective properties against cancer and premature ageing. It may also be essential for the thyroid gland, which controls the body's metabolic rate.

Selenium is found predominantly in wholefoods, seafood and seeds, especially sesame seeds.

Optimal Intake: 100µg
From Diet: 50µg **From Supplements:** 20–100µg

◆ VANADIUM

Vanadium is increasingly being recognised as a mineral which is essential in humans. It is believed to be involved in hormone function, cholesterol metabolism and blood sugar control because it may mimic the action of insulin.

Some research has shown that a deficiency in vanadium may contribute to poor blood sugar control, leading to hypo-glycaemia or diabetes.[4] Animal studies have shown that it improves glucose tolerance, inhibits the formation of choles-terol and improves the laying down of minerals in bones and teeth.[5] Excessive levels of vanadium have been linked to manic depression.

Although there is no RDA for vanadium, an intake of 10–60µg is probably sufficient. The most commonly used form in supplements is vanadyl sulphate.

Good food sources of vanadium include parsley, mushrooms, dill, black pepper and shellfish.

Optimal Intake: 100µg
From Diet: 30µg   **From Supplements:** 25–100µg

♦ ZINC

A large part of the population is at risk of being zinc-deficient – half eat less than 50 per cent of the RDA. Deficiency symptoms are white marks on the nails, lack of appetite or lack of appetite control, pallor, infertility, lack of resistance to infection, poor growth (including hair) and poor skin (including acne, dermatitis and stretch marks), as well as mental and emotional problems. Zinc deficiency plays a role in nearly every major disease including diabetes and cancer: it is needed to make insulin, to boost the immune system and to make the antioxidant enzyme SOD. Zinc is required to make prostaglandins (hormone-like substances) from essential fatty acids which help balance hormones, control inflammation and balance the stickiness of the blood. Sucking zinc lozenges can help to shorten the duration of a cold.

Zinc's main role is the protection and repair of DNA; and for this reason zinc is highest in animals, which have high levels of DNA. The vegetarian diet may therefore be low in zinc. Stress, smoking and alcohol deplete zinc, as does frequent sex, at least for the man, since semen has the highest concentration of zinc in the human body. Oysters are popularly said to be aphrodisiacs – they are also the highest dietary source of zinc and for both the male and female zinc is essential for fertility.

Good food sources of zinc include oysters, lamb, pecan nuts, Brazil nuts, oats, rye and egg yolk.

Optimal Intake: 20mg
From Diet: 7.5mg   **From Supplements:** 10–25mg

3 MULTIMINERAL SUPPLEMENTS

This is one piece of the jigsaw that will make up your personal supplement programme (see page 138)

A good daily multimineral should provide roughly the following levels of minerals.

Boron	1 – 3mg
Calcium	150 – 500mg
Chromium	20 – 100µg
Copper	0.25 – 0.75mg
Iodine	20 – 45µg
Iron	10 – 25mg
Magnesium	75 – 225mg
Manganese	2.5 – 5mg
Molybdenum	20 – 100µg
Selenium	20 – 100µg
Vanadium	25 – 100µg
Zinc	10 – 25mg

chapter 4

The Fats of Life

F‌at is good for you. Eating the right kind of fat is totally essential for optimal health. Essential fats reduce the risk of cancer, heart disease, allergies, arthritis, eczema, depression, fatigue, infections, PMS – the list of symptoms and diseases associated with deficiency is growing every year.

In fact, unless you go out of your way to eat the right kind of fat-rich foods, such as seeds, nuts and fish, the chances are you're not getting enough good fat. Most people in the Western world eat too much of the saturated fats (those that kill) and too little of the essential fats (those that heal).

There are three kinds of fat: saturated, monounsaturated and polyunsaturated. Saturated and monounsaturated fat are not nutrients. You don't need them, although they can be used by the body to make energy. Polyunsaturated fats or oils, however, are essential. Most authorities now agree that, of our total fat intake, no more than one-third should be saturated (hard) fat, and at least one-third should be polyunsaturated oils providing the two essential fats: the linoleic acid family, known as Omega 6; and the alpha-linolenic acid family,

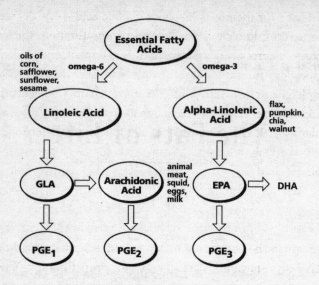

Figure 5 – Omega 3 and 6 fat pathway

known as Omega 3. These two essential fat families also need to be in balance. Most people are deficient in both Omega 6 and Omega 3 fats.

◆ OMEGA 3 – FISH OIL AND FLAX OIL

The modern diet is likely to be more deficient in Omega 3 fats than Omega 6 fats simply because the grandmother of the Omega 3 family, alpha-linolenic acid, and her metabolically active grandchildren, EPA (eicosapentaenoic acid) and DHA (docosahexaenoic acid), are more unsaturated and more prone to damage in cooking and food processing. EPA and DHA can be made into series 3 prostaglandins, which are extremely active hormone-like substances in the body.

As these fats get converted in the body to more 'active' substances, they become more unsaturated and generally the word used for them gets longer (e.g. oleic acid – one degree of unsaturation; linoleic – two degrees of unsaturation; linolenic – three degrees of unsaturation; eicosapentaenoic – five degrees of unsaturation, etc). We can see this increasing complexity as we move up the food chain. For example, plankton, the staple food of small fish, is rich in alpha-linolenic acid. Carnivorous fish, like mackerel or herring, eat the small fish who have converted some of their alpha-linolenic acid to more complex fats. The carnivorous fish continue the conversion. Seals eat them and thus have the highest EPA and DHA concentration. Then Eskimos eat the seals and benefit from the ready-made meal of EPA and DHA, from which they can easily make the series 3 prostaglandins.

These prostaglandins are essential for proper brain function, affecting vision, learning ability, co-ordination and mood. They also help reduce the stickiness of blood, control blood cholesterol and fat levels, improve immune function and metabolism, reduce inflammation and maintain water balance. Symptoms of deficiency include dry skin, inflammatory health problems, water retention, tingling in the arms or legs, high blood pressure or high triglycerides, infections, poor memory and learning problems, lack of co-ordination, impaired vision, and poor growth in children.

The best food sources for Omega 3 fats are fish and flax seeds (also known as linseed). Flax seeds and their oil are less powerful than fish oil (which is already rich in EPA and DHA), because they have to be converted into these by the body. Therefore, you need relatively more to achieve the same effect. In practical terms you need the equivalent of either a flat table-spoon of flax seeds, or a dessertspoon of flax seed oil, which is also available in capsules as a supplement. Supplements usually provide 500 or 1000mg of the oil.

Fish and fish oils provide more powerful sources of the Omega 3 fats, EPA and DHA. Eating fish or their oils bypasses the first two conversion stages of alpha-linolenic acid, to provide EPA and DHA. This is why fish eaters like the Japanese have three times the Omega 3 fats in their body fat compared to the average American. Vegans, who eat more seeds and nuts, have twice the Omega 3 level in their body fat compared to the average American.

While cod liver oil has the greatest percentage of Omega 3 fats, the best fish to eat are the oily ones such as mackerel, herring and salmon. An ideal daily intake is in the order of 500–1000mg, or double if you have an inflammatory health problem, cardiovascular disease or a related mental health problem (see Chapter 8). This is equivalent to eating 100g of fish three or four times a week. Alternatively, you can take a supplement of fish oils containing EPA and DHA. A good-quality cod liver oil supplement provides 400mg. The most concentrated supplements provide 700mg per capsule. If you have arthritis, for example, you'd need to take three such capsules a day.

Since not all products list their nutrients in the same way, the easiest way to measure what you are getting is to look at the label and add up the total amount of EPA plus DHA and compare this to these recommended levels. About half of the Omega 3 fats in fish come from EPA and DHA. It is also worth choosing those brands and products that are 'PCB-free'. Unfortunately our oceans, and consequently fish, are polluted with these industrial chemicals. Fish oils can be purified to be PCB-free. Not all supplement companies choose such purified oils because it increases the cost. Choose those that do.

Optimal Intake: 1000mg
From Diet: 500mg   **From Supplements:** 500mg

◆ OMEGA 6 – EVENING PRIMROSE OIL AND BORAGE OIL

The grandmother of the Omega 6 fat family is linoleic acid. Linoleic acid is converted by the body into gamma-linolenic acid (GLA). GLA then gets converted into DGLA (di-homo-gamma-linolenic acid) and from there into prostaglandins. The particular prostaglandins made from these Omega 6 oils are called 'series 1 prostaglandins'. These keep the blood thin, relax the blood vessels, lower blood pressure, help to maintain water balance in the body, decrease inflammation and pain, improve nerve and immune function, and help insulin to work (which is good for blood sugar balance). This is only the short-list. As every year passes, more and more health-promoting functions are being found. Prostaglandins themselves cannot be supplemented as they are very short-lived. Instead we rely on a good intake of Omega 6 fats from which our bodies can make the prostaglandins we need.

Deficiency signs include high blood pressure, PMS or breast pain, eczema, dry skin, dry eyes, inflammatory health problems such as arthritis, diabetes, multiple sclerosis, mental health problems and excessive thirst.

This family of fats comes exclusively from seeds and their oils. The best seed oils are hemp, pumpkin, sunflower, safflower, sesame, corn, walnut, soybean and wheatgerm oil. About half of the fats in these oils comes from the Omega 6 family, mainly as linoleic acid. An optimal intake would be about 1 dessertspoon a day, or 1 tablespoon of ground seeds. Evening primrose oil and borage oil are the richest known sources of GLA and, by supplementing these direct, you need take in less overall oil to get an optimal intake of Omega 6 fats. The ideal intake is around 150mg of GLA a day, or double this if you have a related health problem. This is equivalent to 1500mg of evening primrose oil, or 750mg of high-potency borage oil, probably the equivalent of a capsule a day. Most evening primrose oil capsules come in 500mg strengths, giving 50mg of GLA. Therefore you would need to supplement three to six capsules to achieve optimal amounts.

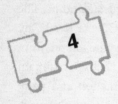

4 ESSENTIAL FATS SUPPLEMENTS

This is one piece of the jigsaw that will make up your personal supplement programme (see page 138)

Essential Balance, available from Higher Nature, and Udo's Oil, available from Savant Distribution Ltd, are two excellent blended seed oils, ideal for use in salad dressings and milk-shakes (see Useful Addresses for suppliers' details).

Optimal Intake (GLA): 150mg
From Diet: 50mg **From Supplements:** 100mg

chapter 5

Energy Nutrients

Numerous nutrients are involved in what is one of the body's most vital functions – to make energy by burning glucose (carbohydrate). This chapter focuses on the B vitamins and chromium (for more on other key players such as vitamin C see Chapters 2 and 7, and for Co-Q10 see Chapter 6).

What you experience as energy, whether mental or physical, is the end result of a process known as catabolism. In a carefully controlled sequence of chemical reactions, food is broken down into its component parts, and these are combusted with oxygen, to make a unit of cellular energy called ATP, which in turn makes muscles work, nerve signals fire and brain cells function. Years ahead of man's primitive attempts to produce energy, this magical process happens inside every single cell of your body and the only waste products are water and carbon dioxide. But, first of all, the fuel has to be refined.

Although we can make energy from protein, fat and carbohydrate, carbohydrate-rich foods are the best kind of fuel. This is because when fat and protein are used to make energy there is a build-up of toxic substances in the body. Carbohydrates are the only 'smokeless' fuel. Our cells require the simplest unit of carbohydrate, glucose. So the first job of the body is to turn all forms of carbohydrate into glucose – this is the ultimate goal of digestion. By eating regularly throughout the day, and avoiding stimulants which rapidly raise blood sugar (sugar, coffee, etc), your cells receive an even supply of energy-giving glucose.

◆ TURNING GLUCOSE INTO ENERGY

Within each of our thirty trillion or so cells – whether it be a muscle, immune or brain cell – exist tiny energy factories called mitochondria (see Figure 6). While the cell's instructions, encoded in DNA, come from both parents, the instructions or DNA within these mitochondria come only from the mother. Whether you like it or not, in this sense you are more like your mother than your father – you inherit the same strengths and weaknesses in the energy-producing department.

If you think this means that all you need to do is eat complex carbohydrates and keep breathing that's only half the story. All these chemical reactions are carefully controlled by enzymes, themselves dependent on no less than eight vitamins and five minerals. Any shortage of these critical catalysts and your energy factories – the mitochondria – go out of tune. The result is inefficient energy production, a loss of stamina, highs and lows – or even just continued lows.

In a survey by the Institute of Optimum Nutrition (ION), 58 per cent of people complained of frequently feeling tired. The researchers found that by simply improving a person's diet and supplementing the many key vitamins and minerals

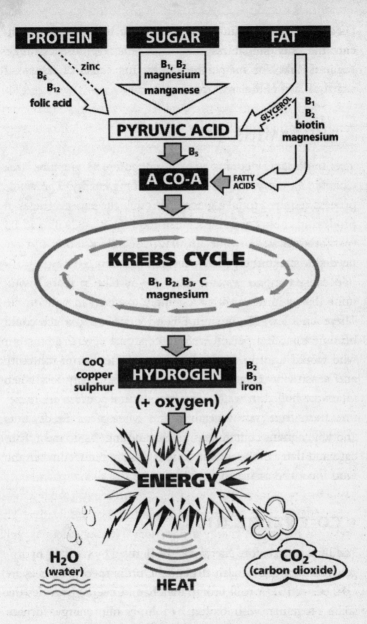

Figure 6 – How mitochondria turn food into energy

needed to turn food into energy, 73 per cent of people experienced a definite improvement in energy. This strongly suggests that, for many, the underlying cause of fatigue is simply a lack of the right nutrients.

◆ B VITAMINS

The important vitamins are the B complex vitamins (see Chapter 2), every one essential for making energy. The whole process required to take glucose through the various stages of producing energy within each cell requires B1, B2, B3 and B5 (pantothenic acid), while B6, B12, folic acid and biotin are needed to make energy from fats and proteins.

Because they are water-soluble, if you take in more B vitamins than you need they are simply excreted in your urine. There are a few, like vitamin B6 and vitamin B3, which could become toxic if a person were to consume several grams but who would want to do that? Because of their water-solubility and sensitivity to heat, B vitamins are also easily lost when foods are boiled in water. The best natural sources are therefore fresh fruit, raw vegetables and wheatgerm. Seeds, nuts and wholegrains contain reasonable amounts, as do meat, fish, eggs and dairy produce. But these levels are reduced when the food is cooked or stored for a long time.

◆ CO-ENZYME Q10

The final stage before energy can be derived by reacting hydrogen with oxygen is also dependent on a special co-enzyme Q10 (Co-Q10). A vital link in the chain, Co-Q10 provides the spark, together with oxygen, to keep our energy furnace burning.

The discovery that Co-Q10 is present in foods, that levels decline with age, and that cellular levels rise when supplements are taken, has led many nutritional scientists to suspect that it may be the missing link in the energy equation. Technically, it cannot be classified as a vitamin since it can be made by the body, even if it isn't made in large enough amounts for optimum health and energy. It is therefore a 'semi-essential' nutrient. (For more on Co-Q10 see Chapter 6.)

◆ ENERGY MINERALS

The minerals iron, calcium, magnesium, chromium and zinc are also vital for making energy. Calcium and magnesium are perhaps the most important because all muscle cells need an adequate supply of these to be able to contract and relax. A shortage of magnesium (very common in people who don't eat much fruit or vegetables) often results in cramps, as muscles are unable to relax.

Magnesium is needed by 75 per cent of the enzymes in your body – and it is vital for carbohydrate metabolism, i.e. the use of carbohydrates to make energy.[6] It is also essential for the transmission of messages between nerve cells. Symptoms of deficiency include things like muscle tremors, muscle weakness, insomnia, nervousness, hyperactivity, depression, confusion, irregular heartbeat, constipation and lack of appetite. Most of these are connected with unbalanced muscle or nerve function.

Zinc, together with vitamin B6, is needed to make the enzymes that digest food which are essential in the process of making energy.[7] They are also required for the production of the hormone insulin, which helps to balance blood sugar levels (blood sugar slumps are a common cause of low energy).

◆ CHROMIUM

The older you are, the less likely you are to be taking in enough chromium – an essential mineral that helps stabilise blood sugar levels. Dr Stephen Davies and colleagues at the Biolab Medical Unit in London analysed 51,665 samples of hair, blood and sweat, taken from 40,872 patients, and found a clear, age-related decline in chromium levels: 75-year-olds had almost half the levels of children aged one to four.[8] This pattern of ever-decreasing chromium is strongly suggestive of a nationwide diet that fails to meet our requirements for this mineral.

Adult diabetics have much lower chromium levels than non-diabetics and, if given chromium, show improved glucose tolerance.[9] Supplementing 200mcg of chromium a day can help even out blood sugar levels, decrease insulin requirement, lower blood cholesterol and triglycerides, and increase cholesterol-removing high-density lipoprotein.[10] The average diet provides only about 30mcg of chromium a day; large amounts are lost when food is refined – 90 per cent from flour, rice or sugar. So only a wholefood diet is likely to provide enough of this essential element, with ideal intakes estimated at 50–200mcg a day. What's more, those with insulin resistance (perhaps due to too much sugar, stimulants or stress) use up chromium at a much faster rate and so become deficient.

Levens of chromium are much higher in wholewheat flour, bread or pasta than in refined products. It is also found in beans, nuts and seeds. Asparagus and mushrooms are especially rich in chromium.

Whether or not you can achieve an optimal intake of chromium from diet alone is debatable. It is therefore wise to take supplements as well as eating wholefoods. The best forms of chromium are either picolinate or polynicotinate. Chromium polynicotinate is chromium bound with niacin (vitamin B3). Although not yet proven, it is thought that chromium may be part of a special molecule produced by the liver, called Glucose Tolerance Factor, whose structure includes chromium, niacin and the amino acids cystine, glycine and glutamic acid.

◆ SUPPLEMENTS FOR ENERGY

Ensuring an optimal intake of all the nutrients involved in turning food into energy is a key part of the energy equation, alongside eating the right kinds of food. One of the easiest ways to guarantee such optimal levels is to take nutritional supplements. Possibly with the exception of Co-enzyme Q10 and chromium, if your need is high, a high-strength multi-vitamin and mineral, plus extra vitamin C, should provide roughly the following levels.

B1 (thiamin)	25–100mg
B2 (riboflavin)	25–100mg
B3 (niacin)	50–150mg
B5 (pantothenic acid)	50–300mg
B6 (pyridoxine)	50–250mg
B12 (cyanocobalamin)	5–100mcg
Folic acid	50–400mcg
Co-enzyme Q10	10–90mg
Vitamin C	1000–3000mg
Calcium	150–600mg
Magnesium	100–300mg
Iron	10–25mg
Zinc	10–25mg
Chromium	20–300mcg

chapter 6

Anti-Ageing Antioxidants

Many substances act as antioxidants in the body. In addition to those covered below, one of the most powerful is vitamin C (which is discussed in much more detail in Chapter 7, as are anthocyanidins). Selenium and zinc are also important antioxidants (for more on their benefits see Chapter 3).

During the last decade more and more research has confirmed that many of the most common twentieth-century diseases are associated with a deficiency of antioxidant nutrients, and can be helped by taking antioxidant supplements. These diseases include Alzheimer's, cancer, cataracts, cardiovascular disease, diabetes, hypertension, infertility, eye problems, measles, mental illness, gum disease, respiratory tract infections and rheumatoid arthritis.

◆ ANTIOXIDANTS IN AGEING

Slowing down the ageing process is no longer a mystery. The best results have consistently been achieved by giving animals low-calorie diets, high in antioxidant nutrients – in other words exactly what they need and no more. This reduces 'oxidative stress' and ensures maximum antioxidant protection. Animals fed in this way not only live up to 40 per cent longer, but they are also more active. Although long-term studies have yet to be completed, there is every reason to assume that the same principles apply to us. Already, large-scale surveys show that the risk of disease and premature death is substantially reduced in those with either high blood levels of antioxidants or high dietary intakes. The main players are vitamins A, C and E, plus beta-carotene (the precursor of vitamin A found in fruits and vegetables), the minerals zinc and selenium, plus glutathione, lipoic acid and Co-Q10. Their presence in your diet, and levels in your blood, may prove the best markers yet of your power to delay death and prevent disease.

◆ WHAT IS AN ANTIOXIDANT?

Oxygen is the basis of all plant and animal life. It is our most important nutrient, needed by every one of our cells every second of every day. Without it we cannot release the energy in food to activate any of our body processes (see Chapter 5). There is one problem though – oxygen is chemically reactive and highly dangerous. In normal biochemical reactions oxygen can become unstable and capable of 'oxidising' neighbouring molecules. This can lead to cellular damage which triggers cancer, inflammation, arterial damage and ageing. Known as 'free oxidising radicals', this equivalent of 'nuclear waste' must be disarmed to remove the danger.

Free radicals are produced by all combustion processes including smoking, exhaust fumes, radiation, fried or barbecued food and normal body processes. Chemicals capable of disarming free radicals are called 'antioxidants'. Some are known essential nutrients, like vitamins A and beta-carotene, C and E. Others, though not essential (bioflavonoids, anthocyanidins, pycnogenol and over 100 other recently identified protectors found in common foods), are very powerful.

The balance between your intake of antioxidants and your exposure to free radicals may literally be the difference between life and death. You can tip the scales in your favour by making simple changes to your diet and taking antioxidant supplements.

◆ ANTIOXIDANTS WORK IN SYNERGY

None of these nutrients works in isolation in the body, nor are people ever deficient in just one nutrient. As good as the results discussed so far appear, they underestimate the power of optimum nutrition in preventing and reversing the ageing, degeneration and cancer processes.

Vitamin C, which is water-soluble, and vitamin E, fat-soluble, are synergistic: together they can protect the tissues and fluids in the body. What's more, when vitamin E has 'disarmed' a carcinogen, it can be reloaded by vitamin C, so their combined presence in the diet and the body has a synergistic effect.

The same is true of selenium and vitamin E. When these nutrients are provided together, the level of cancer protection is considerably multiplied. For example, a study from Finland, carried out by Dr Jukka Salonen and colleagues at the University of Kuopio on 12,000 people over several years, found that those in the top third of both vitamin E and selenium blood levels had a 91 per cent decreased risk of cancer

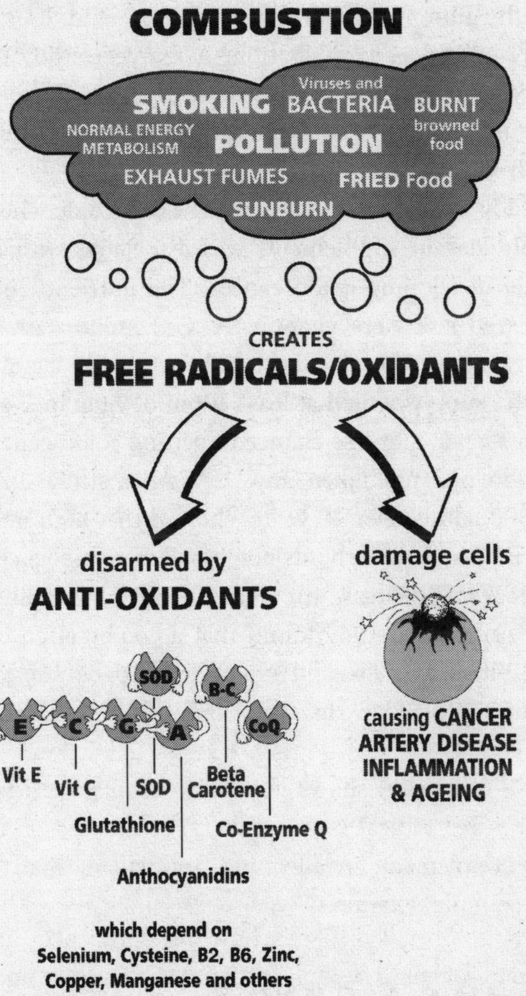

COMBUSTION

SMOKING Viruses and BACTERIA BURNT browned food

NORMAL ENERGY METABOLISM POLLUTION

EXHAUST FUMES FRIED Food

SUNBURN

CREATES

FREE RADICALS/OXIDANTS

disarmed by
ANTI-OXIDANTS

damage cells

causing **CANCER
ARTERY DISEASE
INFLAMMATION
& AGEING**

SOD B-C

E C G A CoQ

Vit E Vit C SOD Beta Carotene

Glutathione Co-Enzyme Q

Anthocyanidins

which depend on
Selenium, Cysteine, B2, B6, Zinc,
Copper, Manganese and others

Figure 7 – Free radicals and antioxidants

compared to those in the bottom third.[11] By having high levels of both these nutrients their risk was less than one-tenth of those with sub-optimal levels. Vitamin C and E is also a powerful anti-cancer combination. A ten-year study on over 11,000 people, completed in 1996, found that those supplementing both vitamin C and vitamin E halved their overall risk of death from all cancers.[12]

One study in Seattle, involving over 800 people who took a daily multivitamin supplement, was associated with halving the risk of developing colon cancer. The nutrients linked to the decreased risk were vitamins A, C, E, folic acid and the mineral calcium. The strongest link was with vitamin E – people who supplemented at least 200iu of vitamin E over ten years had 57 per cent less chance of getting colon cancer than people who had not taken any.[13] Another study, involving over 10,000 adults over 19 years, showed that high intakes of vitamins E, C and carotenoids combined were associated with a 68 per cent decrease in the risk of developing lung cancer.[14] An animal study found that a combination of beta-carotene, vitamins E, C and glutathione to be substantially more cancer-protective than any one of these nutrients in isolation.[15]

Figure 8 (opposite) shows how antioxidants work together to disarm a free radical (an oxidant). For this reason it is far better to supplement an all-round antioxidant than to just take, for example, vitamin C.

◆ VITAMINS A, C AND E

Conversely, a lower level of vitamin A and vitamin E is associated with Alzheimer's disease. Sufferers have half the blood levels of vitamin E and beta-carotene of those people who do

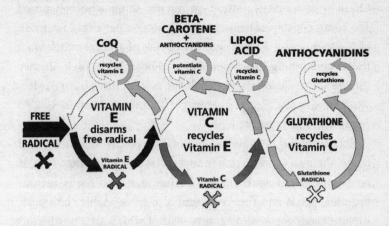

Figure 8 – The synergistic action of antioxidants

not have Alzheimer's.[16] Elderly people with low blood levels of vitamin C have 11 times the risk of developing cataracts compared to those with high blood levels of vitamin C.[17] Similarly, those with low vitamin E blood levels have almost double the risk, while people consuming 400iu of vitamin E a day have half the risk of developing cataracts.[18]

Levels of vitamin A are consistently found to be low in those with lung cancer. In fact, having a low vitamin A level doubles your risk.[19] Similarly, a high intake of beta-carotene from raw fruits and vegetables reduces the risk of lung cancer in non-smoking men and women.[20] In one study supplementing beta-carotene (30mg per day) resulted in improvements in 71 per cent of patients with oral pre-cancer (leukoplakia), while 57 per cent of patients given 200,000iu of vitamin A a day had complete remission.[22]

In relation to heart disease, supplementing vitamin E and

vitamin C effectively halves the risk of ever having a heart attack – in a massive study on nurses, those who consumed 15–20mg per day of beta-carotene had a 40 per cent lower risk of a stroke and a 22 per cent lower risk of a heart attack than those consuming 6mg per day.[22] Those with high dietary intakes of beta-carotene had half the risk of death from cardio-vascular disease. Supplementing 1000mg of vitamin C also reduces blood pressure.[23]

Beta-carotene is found in red/orange/yellow vegetables and fruits. Vitamin C is also rich in vegetables and fruits eaten raw, as heat rapidly destroys it. Vitamin E is found in 'seed' foods, including nuts, seeds and their oils, and also in vegetables like peas, broad beans, corn, wholegrains – all of which are classified as seed foods. Eating sweet potatoes, carrots, watercress, peas and broccoli frequently is a great way to increase your antioxidant levels, provided, of course, that you don't fry them.

Another great antioxidant food is watermelon. The flesh is high in beta-carotene and vitamin C, while the seeds are high in vitamin E and antioxidant minerals zinc and selenium. You can make a great antioxidant cocktail by pulversing the flesh and seeds using a blender or food processor. Seeds and seafood are the best all-round dietary sources of selenium and zinc.

◆ ZINC AND SELENIUM

Discussed more fully in Chapter 3, zinc and selenium are two key antioxidant minerals. This is because they are needed to activate two key antioxidant enzymes: glutathione peroxidase, which is selenium-dependent; and superoxide dismutase, which is dependent on zinc and, to a lesser extent, copper and manganese. Another antioxidant enzyme, catalase, is dependent on iron. However, too much iron can also increase oxidation so you don't want either too much or too little.

♦ Co-Q10

Co-enzyme Q10 (Co-Q10) is not classified as a vitamin because it can be made in the body. Co-Q10 is a vital antioxidant which helps to protect cells from carcinogens and also helps to recycle vitamin E. It is particularly important because of its ability to improve the cells' use of oxygen (for more on this see Chapter 5). In the final and most significant stage of catabolism, when hydrogen is released during the Krebs cycle to react with oxygen, the actual reaction occurs at an atomic level. The components of these elements – electrons – are passed from one atom to the next in what is called the electron transfer pathway. These electrons, which are tiny charged particles, are highly reactive and need to be very carefully handled. They are like nuclear fuel – a potent but very dangerous energy source. Co-Q10 works by controlling the flow of oxygen, making the production of energy more efficient; it also prevents damage caused by these free radicals.

There is evidence that Co-Q10 levels are lower in people with cancer than those without and that people's need for it increases when they have the disease.[24] For this reason, researchers are now studying the effects of giving extra Co-Q10 to combat cancer. The first cases to be reported are of women with breast cancer treated in Denmark. Out of 36 women classified as 'high risk', as their tumours had spread, six patients showed 'apparent partial remission' following the supplementation of 90mg of Co-Q10, together with other antioxidants.[25] An additional three women, treated with 390mg of Co-Q10, had also shown apparent remission.[26]

These results are encouraging and highlight the potential importance of supplementing this nutrient to ensure optimal levels. It is also beneficial in the treatment of cardiovascular disease. No studies have reported toxicity of Co-Q10 even at extremely high doses taken over many years. There is no reason to think that continued supplementation with Co-Q10, as is advised for many vitamins, should have anything but extremely positive results.

Co-Q exists in many foods but not always in a form that we can make use of. There are many different types of Co-Q, from Co-Q1 up to Co-Q10. Yeast, for example, contains Co-Q6 and Co-Q7. Only Co-Q10 is found in human tissue. It is this form that is effective in the ways described above and it is the only form that should be supplemented. However, we can utilise 'lower' forms of Co-Q and convert them into Co-Q10. This conversion process, which occurs in the liver, allows us to make use of the Co-Q found in almost all foods.

But in some people, especially the elderly, the ability to convert lower forms of Co-Q into the active Co-Q10 is impaired or non-existent. Exactly why and to what extent this occurs is not known at the present time. But for these people, Co-Q10 is effectively an essential nutrient. In other words, the body needs to be given a supply of it as opposed to being able to make it, which is probably why so many people are deficient in it.

Some foods contain relatively more Co-Q10, and these foods are our best dietary sources of Co-Q. These include all meat and fish (especially sardines), eggs, spinach, broccoli, alfalfa, potato, soya beans and soya oil, wheat (especially wheatgerm), rice bran, buckwheat, millet, and most beans, nuts and seeds.

Today many supplement companies produce Co-Q10 products. The ideal dosage is 10–90mg a day. It is best absorbed in an oil-soluble form.

◆ GLUTATHIONE, CYSTEINE AND N-ACETYL CYSTEINE

The amino acids cysteine and glutathione also act as antioxidants. Cysteine is often supplemented as N-acetyl-cysteine; the body can use cysteine to make glutathione which is the key ingredient in the antioxidant enzyme, glutathione peroxidase, which is itself dependent on selenium. This enzyme helps to detoxify the body, protecting against car exhaust, carcinogens, infections, excessive alcohol and toxic metals. White meat, tuna, lentils, beans, nuts, seeds, onions and garlic are particularly rich in cysteine and glutathione and have been shown to boost the immune system as well as increase antioxidant power.

Glutathione is not a vitamin, but deserves attention as it is perhaps the most important antioxidant within cells and has proven to be highly cancer-protective. It is like a protein, made out of three amino acids; as well as being an antioxidant in its own right, it is also part of key antioxidant enzymes such as glutathione peroxidase and glutathione transferase. It can also recycle vitamin C, thereby multiplying its ability to promote your health. Glutathione plays a major role in detoxifying the body and counteracting the harmful effects of carcinogens, especially oxidants and radiation, as well as protecting DNA and cell growth.[27] It is a highly effective all-round anti-ageing, anti-degeneration, anti-cancer agent.

Recent studies indicate that glutathione may have an important role to play in both the prevention and treatment of cancer, as it helps to kill cancer cells by improving the body's natural immunity.[28] Glutathione is normally made in the body from the amino acid cysteine which is found in a variety of foods, especially garlic. Supplementing it on its own is mildly effective, but the problem is that the glutathione sacrifices itself to protect the body from oxidants. Glutathione is already included in several chemotherapy drugs.

The recent discovery that glutathione is effectively recycled by anthocyanidins (see below), found in grapes, berries and beetroot, led to a new anti-cancer approach of combining glutathione with anthocyanidins, thereby substantially increasing the power of this key antioxidant.[29] Human trials are now under way, using a supplement called Recancostat Compositum, available in Germany, and early results are encouraging. One trial involves 11 people with advanced colorectal cancer, who had completed two chemotherapy treatments and were given little chance of survival.[30] Three died early in the trial. Of the remaining eight, four have shown remarkable improvement. All are continuing with this potentially important therapy, which has proven to be non-toxic.

◆ ANTHOCYANIDINS

Anthocyanidins, from the flavonoid family, are powerful antioxidants found in a wide variety of foods. They account for the different colours of many plants – for example, purple, red, orange, yellow and green plants all contain different types of anthocyanidins. (So you can be sure of a good intake by eating a naturally colourful diet.)

A diet rich in fruit and vegetables can deliver up to a gram of these important nutrients which may be as significant in their health-promoting properties as vitamins and minerals.

Anthocyanidins (sometimes called anthocyans) provide dramatic colours in foods such as those in black grapes, blueberries and cranberries. They are found in fruits, stems, bark, leaves and, more specifically, in flowers. Grape seeds, bilberries, cranberries and pine bark (pycnogenol) are especially rich sources. Other sources include hibiscus flowers, poppy flowers, cornflowers, mallow flowers, peony flowers, rose leaves and hollyhocks – many of these have traditional uses as natural remedies. A sub-family of the anthocyanidin family – proanthocyanidins – are also found in fruits, roots and shrubs and cover the spectrum of red–violet–blue. Grapes are a rich source of a proanthocyanidin called catechin.

As well as being important antioxidants, anthocyanidins are also anti-inflammatory which can make them useful in treating or preventing a wide range of inflammatory diseases, from asthma to eczema and arthritis. They also help stabilise collagen (our intercellular glue) which protects against ageing, and keeps tissue firm, supple and healthy. One of their most remarkable properties is that they provide protection from a wide variety of toxins in both the watery and fatty parts of the body (unlike vitamin C which protects only the watery parts and vitamin E which works only on fat-based compounds). Much reasearch has demonstrated that, in the laboratory, anthocyanidins can be 50 times stronger than vitamin E.[31] They are even more powerful when combined with other key antioxidants, especially glutathione-related compounds, which they help recycle (see above).

The heart disease prevention power of flavonoids such as anthocyanidins is well illustrated by what is known as the French paradox. Despite smoking, drinking alcohol and eating a high-fat diet, the French have significantly lower rates of heart disease. This led to the theory that drinking wine was protective. A study in Israel proved that red wine reduces oxidation of fats in the blood while white wine increases it.[32] Of course, while alcohol per se has many negative qualities, red wine is especially rich in proanthocyanidins, which almost certainly explains the association between a decreased risk of cardiovascular disease and an increased intake of wine. An alternative and more beneficial strategy would be to drink grape juice or take in another concentrated source of proan-thocyan-idins.

There are two ways to increase your intake of health-promoting anthocyanidins. One is to eat them; the other is to supplement your diet with concentrated extracts. To do both confers the most health benefits. Foods to eat include all sorts of berries, black grapes, citrus fruits, buckwheat and flowers used for herb teas. Drink berry juice and red grape juice (diluted due to its high sugar content) and choose red wine in preference to white. In terms of supplements, many antioxi-dant formulas now include some source of anthocyanidins, together with other vitamins, minerals and substances such as lipoic acid. Supplements of anthocyanidins are likely to name the source. For example, bilberry extract would be in a concentrated form to provide a particular percentage of actual anthocyanidins. So, 100mg of bilberry in a 4:1 concentrate, for example, would provide 25mg of anthocyanidins.

◆ LIPOIC ACID

This is a sulphur-containing vitamin-like substance which has very effective antioxidant properties. It is sometimes known as thioctic acid and plays an important role in the conversion of carbohydrates to energy. As an antioxidant, it is particularly useful because, like anthocyanidins, it is one of the few that is both water- and fat-soluble which means it can protect a wider range of molecules than, say, just vitamin C or vitamin E. In Germany, lipoic acid is an approved drug for the treatment of diabetic neuropathy (a condition which affects the nerves of diabetic people) and, in one study, it was shown to improve the levels of various beneficial substances in the blood of HIV-infected people.[33] Foods said to be high in lipoic acid are liver and yeast. Because of the chemical structure of lipoic acid, it is particularly easy to absorb in either a capsule or tablet form. As a general antioxidant support, a dose of 20–50mg is recommended.

 # 5 ANTIOXIDANT SUPPLEMENTS

This is one piece of the jigsaw that will make up your personal supplement programme (see page 138)

Given the unquestionable value of increasing your antioxidant status, it is wise to make sure that your daily supplement programme contains significant quantities of antioxidants, especially if you are older, live in a polluted city or have any other unavoidable exposure to free radicals.

The easiest way to do this is to take a comprehensive antioxidant supplement, in addition to a good multivitamin and mineral. Most reputable supplement companies produce formulas containing a combination of the following nutrients – vitamin A, beta-carotene, vitamin E, vitamin C, zinc, selenium, glutathione and cysteine, plus plant-based antioxidants such as anthocyanidins from a source such as bilberry or pycnogenol. The total supplementary intake (which may come in part from a multivitamin and extra vitamin C) to aim for is shown overleaf:

A (retinol/beta-carotene)	2500 – 6600µgRE (7500–20,000iu)
Glutathione (reduced)	25 – 75mg
E	66 – 660mg (100–1000iu)
C	1000 – 3000mg
Co-Q10	10 – 50mg
Lipoic acid	10 – 50mg
Anthocyanidin source	50 – 250mg

chapter 7

Immune Boosters

O ur immune strength is totally dependent on the nutrients we take in. Deficiencies in vitamins A, B1, B2, B6, B12, folic acid, C and E suppress immunity, as do deficiencies of iron, zinc, magnesium and selenium. An optimal intake of these nutrients is vital in boosting immune strength. Vitamins B1, B2 and B5 have mild immune-boosting effects compared with vitamin B6. The production of antibodies, so critical in fighting any infection, depends upon B6. The functioning of T cells (vital soldiers in the immune army) also depends on adequate B6 levels. The ideal daily intake is probably 50–100mg. Two other important B vitamins are B12 and folic acid. Both appear essential for proper B-cell and T-cell function. B6, zinc and folic acid are all needed in the rapid production of new immune cells to engage an enemy. All these nutrients are discussed in Chapters 2 and 3.

Since no nutrients work in isolation, it's good to supplement a high-strength multivitamin and mineral. The combination of nutrients even at modest levels can have a strong effect on boosting immunity. Dr Chandra and colleagues, in a research study published in the *Lancet*, gave either a multivitamin and mineral or a placebo to 96 healthy elderly people. Those on the supplement had fewer infections, a stronger immune system (as measured by blood test determination of immune factors), and were generally healthier than those on the placebo.[34]

The nutrients worth adding at large amounts to fight off an infection are the antioxidants and particularly vitamin C, zinc, anthocyanidins (see Chapter 6) and the herbs cat's claw and echinacea.

◆ VITAMIN C

In truth, a whole book could be written about vitamin C and its effects on the immune system. There is no question that more vitamin C means better immune function. These are some of its key roles in boosting your immunity:

◆ Vitamin C is strongly anti-viral. Many viruses, such as flu and the common cold, do not necessarily enter the bloodstream; rather they spread in the mucus on the respiratory tract membranes. Vitamin C has proved successful against every virus tested so far, from HIV to the common cold.[35]

◆ It increases the production of T lymphocytes (important in the immune system).

◆ Vitamin C is needed for a special kind of cell division which results in a rapid increase of both B and T lymphocytes. The flu virus works by depressing this type of cell division.

◆ Infected cells with sufficient vitamin C produce more interferon. This blocks the synthesis of viral proteins, preventing the infected cells from being replicated.

- Vitamin C can be either bacteriostatic or bactericidal (i.e. it can hinder the growth of or kill bacteria, depending on the bug).

- Production of a substance called C3 complement is improved with vitamin C, and this in turn triggers B lymphocytes to manufacture more antibodies or anti-toxins.

- It stimulates a substance called non-lysozyme anti-bacterial factor (NLAF), found in tears, which is of particular importance for people who often suffer from eye infections.

- Vitamin C helps the function of phagocytes, which are cells that gobble up bacteria and other 'rubbish'. They can only work if they contain at least 20mcg of vitamin C per 100 million cells.

- Vitamin C detoxifies, partially at least, many bacterial toxins (which often cause all the unpleasant symptoms), depending on the bug.

- Apart from stimulating natural anti-bacterial factors in the body, vitamin C can also improve the performance of antibiotics.

- Mononuclear phagocytes, a special type of white blood cell, use vitamin C with hydrogen peroxide and some minerals, especially zinc compounds, to kill the invaders that they have captured. In people who are vitamin C deficient, bacteria can be engulfed but cannot be digested or destroyed. Research shows that zinc has a role to play in the prevention of colds, especially if sucked slowly with vitamin C.

- Vitamin C also helps sore eyes and runny nose, as it is a natural antihistamine.

Although an ideal daily intake of vitamin C is 500–3000mg, for anyone fighting an infection or immune-related disease much larger amounts, up to 20,000mg a day, may be taken. The best way to do this is to buy pure ascorbic acid (vitamin C) powder, dissolve it in some juice and water, and drink it throughout the day, thereby keeping the body permanently saturated in this powerful immune-boosting nutrient. Some people prefer the more alkaline form of vitamin C, known as ascorbate (e.g. calcium ascorbate or magnesium ascorbate), as it is less acidic. Always remember to take it with a lot of fluid and to decrease the intake gradually when the infection has passed, rather than to stop suddenly. If you take too much vitamin C you'll get loose bowels which is a sign that you should reduce the dose.

◆ ZINC

Zinc deficiency causes shrinking of the thymus (the master gland that makes T cells and is a key component of our immune system) possibly due to the fact that zinc is needed for release of vitamin A from the liver, which is needed for normal thymus activity. Zinc is also required to produce the enzymes that help eliminate routinely produced cancer cells (not for the large amounts that are produced once cancer is established). The hormone thymulin, which is necessary for T-cell maturation, is also zinc-dependent. The mineral zinc, in doses of 100mg a day, has proved to be anti-viral and is available in lozenges for coughs and colds.[36] This level is for short-term use only.

Seminal fluid is high in zinc, so men with high levels of sexual activity need more of this vital mineral. Deficiency shows up as white spots in the nails, and a decline in the senses of taste and smell.

◆ OTHER MINERALS FOR IMMUNITY

CALCIUM

The mineral calcium is vital for the immune system. It is needed by all phagocytic cells in order to perform their job of attaching to and gobbling up foreign material. Cytotoxic T cells need calcium in order to make the enzymes which they produce to kill foreign cells. Complement proteins – which help destroy unwanted material – cannot join together to become active without calcium. It is needed to destroy viruses and to generate fever, which enhances the role of macrophages.

MAGNESIUM

Calcium works with magnesium which is no less important for immunity: it is vital for antibody production, the thymus and much more. Deficiency can cause a rise in histamine levels and hence increase allergic reactions.

IRON

The right amount of iron boosts overall resistance to infection, but too much is actually bad for the immune system. Iron found in food has low toxicity, so iron-rich foods (such as meat, eggs, green vegetables and dried fruit) are generally preferable to supplements. Vitamin C enhances absorption of iron from food.

Iron is essential for the production of antibodies, white blood cells and enzymes made by some of the body's immune army cells. It is needed for the detoxification of some drugs and bacterial toxins. Bacteria, however, need iron for reproduction, so it is wise to avoid iron in supplements or iron-rich foods when suffering from a bacterial infection. When you have a bacterial infection, white blood cells produce an iron-binding protein to tie it up, so there is no sense in overworking the system at this time.

SELENIUM

Selenium helps in the production of antibodies. Research on animals has shown that there is no antibody production at all when animals are deprived of vitamin E and selenium. It has been suggested that these two, given at the time of vaccination, could increase antibody production and hence the effectiveness of the vaccine. Selenium also helps to produce an important antioxidant enzyme, glutathione peroxidase (see Chapter 6). Without this mineral, white blood cells lose their efficiency in recognising invaders.

◆ CAT'S CLAW

Uncaria tomentosa or cat's claw (its thorn is shaped like the claw of a cat) is a woody vine that can wind its way over 30 metres up through the trees in its attempt to reach light in the Peruvian rainforests. The native Indians have long used its bark to treat cancer, joint problems and many other diseases.

Although research is still young, it has been so convincing that the plant has become an endangered species and in 1989 the Peruvian government banned the harvesting and use of the root of the two main species (*U. tomentosa* and *U. guianensis*). It appears that the bark contains most or all of the medicinal properties. It grows back after harvesting, whereas cutting or damaging the whole root kills the entire plant. It is still feared that worldwide demand for this bark exceeds production so, as with ginseng, the purchaser needs to be aware of non-therapeutic substitutes. You can guard against this by purchasing cat's claw from reputable suppliers such as Higher Nature or Solgar (see Useful Addresses).

Components of cat's claw have been shown to increase the ability of white blood cells to carry out phagocytosis (i.e. to engulf, digest and so destroy an invading germ).

It has also been shown to contain other chemicals which reduce inflammation. It is potentially a super-plant with immune-stimulating, antioxidant, anti-inflammatory, anti-tumour and anti-microbial properties.

Austrian researchers have also identified extracts of cat's claw which they have been using to treat cancer and viral infections. One problem they have come across is that different samples contain different amounts of these therapeutic chemicals, which makes dosage difficult to calculate; it is not yet known whether this is due to location, seasonal or species variation.

Cat's claw comes either as capsules, with 2g being a good daily dose, or as tea (loose or in teabags). A 2g dose is probably equivalent to two cups a day. You can get more out of the loose tea by boiling it for five minutes and then adding a little blackcurrant and apple juice concentrate to improve the taste.

◆ ECHINACEA

This root of the plant *Echinacea purpurea* is probably the most widely used immune-boosting herb. It possesses interferon-like properties and is an effective anti-viral agent against flu and herpes.[37] It contains special kinds of polysaccharides, such as inulin, which increase macrophage production. These have been shown to destroy cancer cells in the test tube and fight off the undesirable yeast *Candida albicans*.[38]

But echinacea isn't just something to take when you've got an infection. One study on a group of healthy men found that after five days of taking 30 drops of echinacea extract three times a day, their white blood cells had doubled their 'phagocytic' power.[39] Whether echinacea's immune-boosting properties are maintained over a long period of time is not yet known. Some researchers recommend just using these herbs to boost immunity when your health is actually under threat.

When you're fighting an infection, echinacea is best taken either as capsules of the powdered herb (2000mg a day) or as drops of concentrated extract (20 drops three times a day).

◆ ELDERBERRY

Berries are extremely good for the immune system as they contain high levels of antioxidants including anthocyanidins (see Chapter 6). But elderberries have an extra-special property, discovered by a virologist Madeleine Mumcuoglu, working with Dr Jean Linderman, who first identified interferon.

For a virus to take hold it must first get into the body cells, which it does by puncturing their walls with tiny spikes made of haemagglutinin. 'Viral spikes are covered with an enzyme called neuraminidase, which helps break down the cell wall,' says Mumcuoglu. 'The elderberry inhibits the action of that enzyme. My guess is that we'll find elderberry acts against viruses in other ways as well.'

In a double-blind controlled trial in Israel, researchers tested the effects of Sambucol (a specially prepared extract of elderberry) in people diagnosed with any one of a number of strains of the influenza virus. Their results, published in the *Journal of Alternative and Complementary Medicine*, showed a significant improvement in symptoms – fever, cough, muscle pain – in 20 per cent of patients within 24 hours, and in a further 73 per cent of patients within 48 hours. After three days 90 per cent had achieved complete relief of symptoms, compared to those on the placebo who took at least six days to recover.[40]

While this is only the first published trial of elderberry extract, the results to date are very encouraging. Sambucol, which comes as a liquid extract, is available in the UK from healthfood stores.

6 IMMUNE-BOOSTING SUPPLEMENTS

This is one piece of the jigsaw that will make up your personal supplement programme (see page 138)

It is well worth taking an all-round supplement on an ongoing basis to keep your immune system on top form. The levels given below are recommended as protective doses, and should be stepped up dramatically when your immune system is actually fighting off any infection or illness. For more information on how to do that, see my book *Boost Your Immune System*, co-authored with Jennifer Meek (see Recommended Reading).

	Prevention	Optimum prevention	Therapeutic
Vitamin C	1000mg	2000mg	3000mg
Anthocyanidins (Bilberry 4:1)	10mg	20mg	30mg
Anthocyanidins (Elderberry 4:1)	10mg	20mg	30mg
Cat's claw extract (3:1)	33.3mg	66.6mg	100mg
Echinacea (3:1)	33.3mg	66.6mg	100mg
Zinc	3mg	6mg	9mg

chapter 8

Memory and Mood Enchancers

Your intelligence and memory aren't purely determined by your genetic programming. Although there is clearly an in-built element to them both, the development of learning skills and what you eat can make a big difference to your mental abilities.

The brain and nervous system – our mental 'hardware' – are made up of a network of neurons, special cells which are each capable of forming tens of thousands of connections with others. Thinking represents a pattern of activity across this network. Such activity, or exchange of signals, involves neurotransmitters, the chemical messengers in the brain. When we learn, we actually program the wiring of the brain. And when we think, we change the activity of neurotransmitters. Since both the brain and neurotransmitters are derived from nutrients in food, it is not surprising that what we eat has a bearing on our mental performance.

In 1986 Gwillym Roberts, a schoolteacher and nutritionist from the Institute for Optimum Nutrition, and David Benton, a psychologist from Swansea University College, decided to

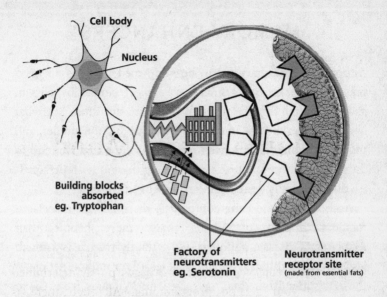

Cell body

Nucleus

Building blocks absorbed eg. Tryptophan

Factory of neurotransmitters eg. Serotonin

Neurotransmitter receptor site (made from essential fats)

Figure 9 – How the brain communicates

investigate whether giving a person an optimal intake of the nutrients that are used by the brain and nervous system would improve intellectual performance. Sixty schoolchildren were put onto either a special multivitamin and mineral supplement designed to ensure an optimal intake of key nutrients or a placebo (dummy pill). On analysing the diets of these school-children before the trial, a significant number were getting less than the RDA level of at least one nutrient. After eight months, the non-verbal IQs of those taking the supplements had risen by over 10 points! No changes were seen in those on the placebos, nor in a control group of students who had taken neither supplements nor placebos.[41] Since this landmark study, 12 further trials have proved the IQ-boosting effects of multivitamin and mineral supplements.

MEMORY ENHANCERS

Although studies have yet to be performed, there is no good reason to assume that adults can't achieve similar benefits in sharpening intelligence through optimum nutrition. But what about sharpening the memory? What about the milder and more commonly experienced memory decline that we tend to ascribe to the normal process of ageing or simply to personality differences? Is there room for improvement here?

According to the drug companies, there is. 'Age-associated memory impairment affects many more people than Alzheimer's disease, although, it's certainly true, it is a much less severe condition. We believe at least four million people in the UK suffer from this,' says Dr Paul Williams from Glaxo Pharmaceuticals, who have been developing drugs to enhance memory and mental performance. According to a report in *The Economist* magazine, 'The American pharmaceutical industry is developing more than 140 types of smart pills in its laboratories, making them the tenth-largest class of drugs being researched.' Even larger than the market for Alzheimer's is the market for the new 'disease' of Age-Associated Memory Decline (AAMD).

For the pharmaceutical industry, the advantage of these drugs is that they are not nutrients but man-made substances (which means that they can be patented after millions of pounds have been spent on research). The disadvantage of such man-made chemicals is that, although modelled on nutrients, they are alien to the human body. They never produce a 'perfect fit' in our enzyme systems and, while creating the desired effect in the short term, in the long term they can knock the body's chemistry out of balance. Of course, with most of these new smart drugs, the long-term effects have yet to be discovered.

There is another, safer way to enhance your memory, mind and mood – and that is to ensure that you take in optimal levels of the nutrients from which your body can make key brain chemicals, through your diet and in supplements.

◆ CHOLINE AND DMAE

Perhaps the key brain chemical for memory is acetylcholine, a neurotransmitter derived from the nutrient choline. Fish, especially sardines, are rich in choline – hence the old wives' tale about fish being good for the brain. Acetylcholine is partly responsible for the way we connect sensory information with memories and then respond appropriately. However, you don't simply make more acetylcholine by eating choline; vitamin B5 is essential for the formation of acetylcholine in the body. Some forms of choline cross more easily from the blood into the brain – such as phosphatidyl choline and a precursor for choline called DMAE (short for dimethylaminoethanol) which accelerates the brain's production of acetylcholine.

While both of these substances can be made by the brain and are therefore not classified as essential nutrients, there is evidence that supplementing DMAE has positive effects on memory and learning. Slight chemical variations of DMAE have been marketed as the drug Deaner or Deanol, which have proven highly effective in helping those with learning problems, attention deficit disorder, memory and behaviour problems. DMAE is also found naturally in fish.

◆ PYROGLUTAMATE

Another key brain chemical that appears to enhance memory and mental function is the amino acid pyroglutamate and its derivatives, which are highly concentrated in the human brain and spinal fluid. In fact, so powerful are its effects that there are now many slight variations of this key brain chemical being marketed as drugs for learning- and memory-related problems such as Alzheimer's.

Numerous studies using these 'smart drugs' have shown that they enhance memory and mental function, not only in those with pronounced memory decline but also in people with so-called normal memory function.[42] Animal research suggests that pyroglutamate may increase the number of receptors for acetylcholine and improve communication between the left and right hemispheres of the brain.[43] While there is still much to learn about exactly how pyroglutamate improves mental function, there is no doubt that it does. Being an amino acid, pyroglutamate is found in many foods, including fish, dairy products, fruit and vegetables.

◆ PHOSPHATIDYL SERINE

Known as 'the memory molecule', phosphatidyl serine (PS) is another smart nutrient that can genuinely boost your brain power. PS is one of the phospholipids which are essential for the health of the liver, immune system, nerves and brain. PS is especially plentiful in the brain and there is increasing scientific evidence that PS supplements improve memory, mood, stress resistance, learning and concentration.

While the body can make its own PS, we rely on receiving some directly from diet, which makes PS a semi-essential nutrient. The trouble is that modern diets are deficient in PS unless you happen to eat a lot of organ meats, in which case you may take in 50mg a day. A vegetarian diet is unlikely to achieve even 10mg a day. The memory-boosting properties of PS are probably due to its ability to help brain cells communicate. Unlike neurotransmitters (which deliver messages from one neuron to another) phosphatidyl serine forms a vital part of the 'docking port' for these messenger molecules, technically known as the receptor site.

PS is particularly helpful for those with learning difficulties or age-related memory decline. In one study by Dr Thomas Crook, published in *Neurology*, vol 41(5) (1991), pp. 644–9, 149 people with age-associated memory impairment were given a daily dose of 300mg of PS or a placebo. When tested after 12 weeks, the ability of those on the PS to match names to faces (a recognised measure of memory and mental function) improved to the equivalent level of people 12 years younger.

◆ OMEGA 3 FATS

Another essential component of the receptor sites for neurotransmitters are Omega 3 fats (see Chapter 4). These essential fats include EPA and DHA and are found mainly in oily fish and also in flax, hemp and walnut oils. DHA is particularly important for mental performance and has an important role in the development of the brain during pregnancy and infancy. It is therefore essential that pregnant women either have a regular dietary source of these Omega 3 fats or supplement them. DHA is highly concentrated in the brain and nervous system and not only improves learning and age-related memory decline but also greatly enhances mood. In one study, people with depression were given 9.6mg of Omega 3 oils and experienced substantial improvement in their manic depression over a four-month period.[44] DHA has also been shown to improve dyslexia and dyspraxia. Dr Jacqueline Stordy from the University of Surrey found that DHA improved the reading ability and behaviour of adults with dyslexia.[45]

An ideal intake of EPA and DHA a day is in the order of 500–1000mg, or double if you have a related mental health problem. This is equivalent to eating 100g of fish (preferably salmon, mackerel, tuna or herring) three or four times a week. Alternatively, you can take a supplement of fish oils containing EPA and DHA. A good-quality cod liver oil supplement can provide up to 400mg. The most concentrated supplements provide 700mg per capsule. If, for example, you had dyslexia, you'd need to take three such capsules a day for maximum effect.

For vegetarians, flax seed oil is the most direct source of Omega 3 fats. In practical terms you need the equivalent of either a flat tablespoon of flax seeds, or a dessertspoon of flax seed oil, which is also available in capsules. You will need to take quite a few of the capsules to make up the equivalent of the actual oil. Supplements usually provide 500mg or 1000mg of the oil per capsule.

◆ GINGKO BILOBA

Gingko biloba is a herbal remedy that has been used for memory enhancement in the East for thousands of years. It comes from one of the oldest species of tree known. Research has shown that it improves short-term and age-related memory loss, slow thinking, depression, circulation and blood flow to the brain.[46] It has also been seen to significantly improve Parkinson's and Alzheimer's diseases over a 12 month period.[47]

Gingko usually comes in capsule form and you should look for a brand that shows the flavonoid concentration, which determines strength. The recommended flavonoid concentration is 24 per cent, of which one would take 120–160mg in two or three divided doses each day. It is suggested that you try the product for between three and six months before evaluating the results.

♦ B VITAMINS

B vitamins have many roles to play in ensuring optimal brain function. B3 (niacin) is particularly good for memory enhancement. In one study 141mg of niacin was given daily to a group of subjects of various ages. Memory was improved by 10–40 per cent in all age groups.[48]

B5 (pantothenic acid) has many functions in the body. It is essential for the brain and helps improve energy. Suggested dosage for memory enhancement is 500–1000mg daily. It is essential for the formation of acetylcholine (see page 00).

B12 has been shown in laboratory experiments to accelerate the rate at which rats learn – it is essential for the health of nerve cells.[49] As it can be hard to absorb, it is suggested that you take 1000mcg daily. Taking B12 in a sublingual (under-the-tongue) formula is even better for absorption.

B6 (pyridoxine) has an important role in brain function, as it is essential for the manufacture of neurotransmitters. It is also necessary for the conversion of amino acids into serotonin (a deficiency in this important neurotransmitter can cause depression and other problems). The section on 5-HTP (below) has more information on serotonin. One study showed that about a fifth of depressed people who took part were deficient in pyridoxine.[50] Suggested supplementation is 50–200mg in divided doses throughout the day.

It is important to remember that B vitamins should be taken in a complex (i.e. all together) and if you wish to concentrate on a specific B vitamin you should take this in conjunction with a lower-dose complex. (For more on B vitamins, including supplementation, see Chapter 2.)

MOOD ENHANCERS

◆ 5-HTP – NATURE'S BLUES-BUSTER

While many of the nutrients discussed above improve memory and mental function, they also help stabilise mood. If you're feeling depressed, you may be deficient in serotonin, a vital brain chemical that helps to keep you in a good mood. It is thought that possibly half of all people with clinical depression have serotonin deficiency, which is much more common in women. Conventional medicine involves the prescription of anti-depressant drugs, like Prozac, that block the breakdown of serotonin, thereby keeping more circulating in the brain. The trouble is that these kinds of drugs have unpleasant side-effects in about a quarter of those who take them and severe reactions in a minority.

The good news is that there is a natural alternative with no side-effects. Instead of blocking the breakdown of serotonin, brain levels can actually be raised by supplementing the substance the body uses to make serotonin. This is called 5-hydroxytryptophan (or 5-HTP for short) and is derived from a plant called *Griffonia simplifica*. Studies have proven that this nutrient is as effective as the best anti-depressants without the side-effects.[51] The recommended dosage is 100mg of 5-HTP, twice a day. Some supplements also provide various vitamins and minerals such as B6, which are needed to turn 5-HTP into serotonin.

◆ ST JOHN'S WORT

St John's wort (*Hypericum perforatum*) is becoming the top natural treatment for mild to moderate depression, with all the benefits of prescription anti-depressants, without the side-effects, at a tenth of the cost. Fifteen medical studies have now shown that it works, in some cases better than drugs.[52] How it works is a bit of a mystery. One of its actions is to stop the body breaking down serotonin, the key brain chemical that controls mood. It also has a mild anti-anxiety effect; it has been shown to aid sleep and can help reduce PMS. For the maximum anti-depressant effect, you need 300mg of a stand-ardised extract containing 0.3 per cent hypericin (the active ingredient) three times a day. Start with two 300mg capsules, then increase to three after a week. Some people report imme-diate improvement, but it usually takes up to three weeks to notice a difference.

 ## 7 MEMORY- AND MOOD-ENHANCING SUPPLEMENTS

This is one piece of the jigsaw that will make up your personal supplement programme (see page 138)

While 5-HTP or St John's wort are worth supplementing if you are prone to depression, a good memory- and mood-enhancing supplement for general use might contain a combination of the following nutrients:

Phosphatidyl choline	250–400mg
Phosphatidyl serine	20–45mg
Vitamin B3 (niacin)	10–15mg
Gingko biloba	20–30mg
Vitamin B12 (cyanocobalamin)	5–10μg
Folic acid	100–200μg
Vitamin B5 (pantothenic acid)	200–300mg
DMAE	200–300mg
Arginine pyroglutamate	300–450mg

chapter 9

The Hormone Helpers

Hormonal problems affect many women and a minority of men. These problems include PMS, menopausal symptoms, fibroids, ovarian cysts, endometriosis, polycystic breast disease and hormone-related cancers, of which cancer of the breast is the most common. Men also experience menopause-like symptoms, known as the andropause, which include loss of sex drive and motivation, weight gain, and enlarged breast tissue. Prostate enlargement and prostate and testicular cancer are also hormone-related conditions which are becoming more common.

Hormones are similar to neurotransmitters (see Chapter 8) in that they act as chemical messengers. They are also made in the body from components taken in from diet. Not surprisingly, hormone-like substances abound in natural foods. However, it is only relatively recently that we have begun to recognise the extent to which foods that are rich in certain phytonutrients influence our hormonal health.

There are a number of ways in which specific food supplements can also help to balance our hormones. Vitamins and minerals, especially vitamins B3, B6, folic acid, biotin, vitamins C and E, zinc and magnesium (see Chapters 2 and 3), help the body to make hormones. And essential fats help the body to 'read' the hormone signals (see Chapter 4).

◆ PHYTO-OESTROGENS

Many foods contain hormone-like substances that affect the body's hormone balance. Oestrogen-like plant compounds are often called phyto-oestrogens (phyto = plant). One might think that eating foods rich in phyto-oestrogens would be bad news. Yet the reverse seems to be true. Soya products, rich in the isoflavones genistein and diadzein, are reputed to protect against breast and prostate cancer, which are notably low among communities with a soya-based diet.

There are two possible explanations for this apparent contradiction. The first is that phyto-oestrogens may lock onto and block the body's oestrogen receptors, thereby making it harder for harmful chemicals to disrupt hormone signals. The second is that these phytonutrients may act more like hormone regulators, rather than simply mimicking oestrogen or progesterone. Since mankind has been exposed to these plant chemicals for millennia, it is highly likely that our bodies have adapted to deal with them in the kinds of quantities we are exposed to from eating natural foods.

While the general consensus is in favour of eating foods rich in these phytonutrients in moderate amounts, there are also grounds for caution. One should not eat vast amounts of phyto-oestrogen-rich foods, especially at key phases of development, such as during pregnancy or early infancy. (Some animals exclusively fed on soya feed have shown symptoms of toxicity.)

Citrus fruit, wheat, alfalfa, hops, oats, fennel, celery and rhubarb all contain phyto-oestrogens. There is a small amount of evidence that these foods may help to balance hormones and could play a part in helping to reduce symptoms associated with hormonal imbalance.[53]

ISOFLAVONES

Soya products and tofu are both excellent sources of isoflavones, which are powerful phyto-oestrogens. Isoflavones are known to decrease the risk of hormone-related cancers, including breast and prostatic cancer.[54] Two particular isoflavones have been identified – genistein and diadzein. An ideal intake for cancer prevention is 100–200mg a day, which is equivalent to a 350g serving of soya milk or a serving of tofu. Tofu, a curd made from the soya bean, is the richest source of isoflavones, while very processed soya products are the poorest source.[55]

You can now buy isoflavones in supplement form. Look on the label for a 'fermented' soya-based product, as these are more potent; and make sure that the active ingredients are in their '-ein' formation not in the '-in' formation. That is, look for 100mg tablets which contain approximately 700mg of genistein (not genestin), 680mg of diadzein (rather than diadzin) and 200mg of glycitein. You can take up to six of these tablets but do start slowly as you may have very good results on less rather than more.

◆ HERBAL REMEDIES

Many herbal remedies are now available as supplements due to their beneficial effects on balancing hormones. The most popular and best proven remedies are shown below. They are best taken under the guidance of a qualified herbalist or clinical nutritionist. You can take the herbs in tea or capsule form – they are widely found in specially blended formulas.

AGNUS CASTUS

The plant *Vitex agnus castus*, also known as chaste tree, has a long history. Traditionally, it has been used to relieve premenstrual and menopausal problems. One study, in which the herb was given to 1542 women, found that 90 per cent reported a significant reduction of PMS symptoms.[56] Agnus castus has the effect of stimulating and normalising the function of the pituitary gland especially by helping to maintain the right progesterone balance. This herb works just as well, whether the person has a hormone excess or deficiency, because it acts as a regulator, helping to stabilise hormonal signals. It has also been shown to stimulate libido, reduce hot flushes, and help improve vaginal dryness, breast tenderness and menstrual cramps. Agnus castus does take some time to work – you may need to take it for 8–12 weeks before you get a result.

BLACK COHOSH

Black cohosh (*Cimicifuga racemosa*), or black snake root, is an old Native American remedy. It contains phyto-oestrogens (see page 104) and is excellent for menopausal problems because it helps to balance female hormones. Black cohosh is also beneficial for painful menstruation, menstrual cramps and trouble-free childbirth. Do not take when menstruating or pregnant.

DONG QUAI AND WILD YAM

These both have progesterone-favourable effects on the body. Yams are especially rich in diosgenin, from which progesterone can be made, but only in the laboratory, not in the human body. We cannot turn these phytonutrients into progesterone itself, so, while these plants may help to balance hormones, they cannot eliminate the need for progesterone in a person who is progesterone-deficient. Both wild yam and dong quai are particularly good for menopausal problems such as sleeplessness, hot flushes and vaginal dryness. Wild yam is also useful for menstrual cramps.

GINSENG AND LICORICE

These are thought to contain quite powerful 'adaptogens' (substances that help restore hormonal balance). For example, licorice appears to increase oestrogen when levels are too low and decrease oestrogen when levels are too high. Both licorice and ginseng support the adrenal hormones and so help protect us from stress.

Ginseng is a classic herbal remedy for increasing one's ability to deal with stress. This is true of both Panax ginseng (Chinese ginseng) and Siberian ginseng (which is actually a different herb altogether). Panax ginseng is particularly good for menopausal problems as it helps to balance the female hormones, especially if oestrogen levels are low. Both have widespread use for a number of hormone-related conditions, probably because adrenal hormones and sex hormones are very closely linked – particularly as the adrenal glands produce small amounts of sex hormones.

Saw palmetto and damiana

These are probably the two most popular herbs for male hormonal health. Saw palmetto gained renown in the treatment of prostatitis (enlargement of the prostate gland), a condition suffered by many men over 40 years old. Damiana, which has a testosterone-like effect, has long been associated with increasing male potency.[57] These herbs, together with ginseng, are often included in male herbal tonics.

8 HORMONE-BALANCING SUPPLEMENTS

This is one piece of the jigsaw that will make up your personal supplement programme (see page 138)

In summary, the inclusion of the right phytonutrient foods and herbs may help the body to adapt, thus restoring and maintaining hormonal balance. Many supplements designed to support female or male health contain combinations of these herbs and are likely to be beneficial.

Female formulae might include, in addition to essential fats, vitamins and minerals:

Agnus castus	250–500mg
Black cohosh	100–200mg
Dong quai	200–400mg
Wild yam	200–400mg
Isoflavones	100–600mg
Ginseng	200–500mg

Male formulae might include, in addition to essential fats, vitamins and minerals:

Damiana	200–400mg
Saw palmetto	100–300mg
Ginseng	300–1000mg

However, if you wish to take large amounts of these herbs it is best to do so under the guidance of a herbalist or clinical nutritionist.

chapter 10

Natural Pain-Killers and Anti-Inflammatories

———

Many disease processes involve inflammation, often characterised by swelling, redness, pain and heat. These include all the 'itis' diseases – arthritis, dermatitis, colitis, nephritis and hepatitis, as well as asthma and others not often associated with inflammation, such as Alzheimer's and Parkinson's in which parts of the brain become inflamed. Inflammation also lies at the root of atherosclerosis, the common cause of thrombosis, heart attacks and strokes. In addition, it is an underlying cause of irritable bowel syndrome, Crohn's disease and ulcerative colitis, now suffered by eight million people in Britain.

Inflammation is the body's way of showing that a person's intake from the environment, including diet, drugs and environmental chemicals, has exceeded their capacity to adapt. Several key areas need to be examined to discover what exactly is contributing to the inflammatory health problem. Often impaired liver detoxification needs to be redressed with diet, herbs and nutrients. Other considerations are disturbed blood sugar control or an imbalance of oxidants vs antioxidants (see

Chapters 5 and 6). Food intolerances or allergies can also be a source of inflammation. Finally, a deficiency or imbalance in essential fatty acids may often lie at the root of inflammation and pain.

There are an increasing number of natural pain-killers and anti-inflammatory agents available, some of which have proved just as effective as drugs but without the side-effects.

◆ ESSENTIAL FATS

The essential fats (or essential fatty acids) effective in decreasing pain and inflammation are the Omega 3 oils EPA and DHA, as well as GLA, the pre-converted essential fat, which is high in evening primrose oil and borage oil. (For more on these fats see Chapter 4.)

Pain and inflammation are often triggered by an imbalance in prostaglandins (short-lived, hormone-like substances in the body, derived from essential fats found in the diet). However, not all prostaglandins trigger pain and inflammation (see Chapter 4). While one group of prostaglandins encourages inflammation (prostaglandin type 2), two other groups of prostaglandins (types 1 and 3) have been shown to reduce inflammation in animals in a variety of studies. Redressing any deficiencies in these essential fats and decreasing your dietary intake of the wrong kinds of fats (i.e. saturated or processed fats) will ensure that these prostaglandins are in the correct ratio, and this can greatly ease inflammation.

EVENING PRIMROSE OIL

Evening primrose oil has proven at least as effective as non-steroidal anti-inflammatory drugs (NSAIDs) in reducing inflammation. In a trial comparing the effects of essential fatty acids with NSAIDs, the results were definitely positive. Arthritic patients, stable on NSAIDs, were assigned to one of three groups. One received 100 per cent evening primrose oil, the other 80 per cent evening primrose oil and 20 per cent fish oil, and the third a placebo (dummy pill). After three months, patients were encouraged to reduce or discontinue their NSAID medication over the next nine months. At the end of this time, everyone was put on placebos. About 90 per cent of those taking essential fatty acids reported improvement and were able to stop, or at least considerably reduce, the NSAIDs, compared to 30 per cent in the placebo group. Almost all who had improved on essential fatty acids regressed when placed on the placebo.[58]

GLA

The amount of GLA required to have this effect is quite high. I recommend 200–300mg GLA per day, reducing to 150mg after three months if inflammation reduces and symptoms stay stable. Only 9–10 per cent of the oil in evening primrose oil is GLA so that means you need to take 3000mg of evening primrose oil, or six 500mg capsules per day. Borage oil contains a higher proportion of GLA and you can get single capsules which provide 250mg of GLA. One of these a day is an essential part of an anti-inflammatory strategy. Supplementing GLA has been shown to be more effective when the co-factor vitamins and minerals (vitamin B6, zinc, B3 and vitamin C) are also supplied.

OMEGA 3 FATS

Even more important for reducing inflammation than GLA are the Omega 3 fats found in oily fish, particularly herring, mackerel, salmon and tuna (see Chapter 4). These fats are derived from an essential oil called linolenic acid, which is found in small amounts in some nuts and seeds. The richest source is flax seed, and its oil.

Studies have also confirmed that supplementing these fish oils can help reduce pain and inflammation. In one study, 17 patients with arthritis were given 1.8g of EPA a day. After 12 weeks they had significantly less stiffness and tenderness of joints. The improvement didn't last when the patients stopped taking the EPA supplements.[59]

These positive results were confirmed by another study in which rheumatoid arthritis patients on NSAID medication were given ten fish oil capsules daily and compared with people on NSAIDs alone. After six weeks there was a significant reduction in the number of painful joints in those taking fish oil, compared to those simply on NSAIDs. When the NSAID medication was withdrawn this improvement vanished, and reduction in pain on the fish oils alone was similar to that on NSAIDs alone.[60] In other words fish oils were as effective as taking NSAIDs.

This strongly suggests that taking in a large enough amount of fish oil is anti-inflammatory – probably due to its EPA and DHA content – and may be as effective as NSAID medication in some cases, without the side-effects. (For more information on supplementation of Omega 3 oils, see page 97.)

◆ CURCUMIN

The bright yellow pigment of the spice turmeric contains the active compound curcumin which has a variety of powerful anti-inflammatory actions – trials in which it was given to arthritic patients have shown it to be similarly effective to the anti-inflammatory drugs, without the side-effects.[61] Like the NSAIDs, it blocks the formation of the pro-inflammatory prostaglandins (PGE2), as well as leukotrienes, another type of inflammatory mediator.[62] It is a powerful antioxidant (see Chapter 6) and has been shown to promote detoxification. Curcumin is highly recommended for easing pain and inflammation in both osteoarthritis and rheumatoid arthritis as well as in post-operative inflammation. An effective dose is 500mg, one to three times a day.

◆ BOSWELLIA

Boswellia serrata, also known as Indian frankincense, is proving to be a very powerful natural anti-inflammatory agent, used mainly for arthritis, without the side-effects of current drugs. The boswellic acid contained within the herb achieves comparative anti-inflammatory effects without the associated gut problems experienced with anti-inflammatory and pain-killing drugs such as aspirin. Boswellic acid appears to reduce joint swelling, restores and improves blood supply to inflamed joints, provides pain relief and improves morning stiffness.

In one study where patients initially received boswellic acid, and then later a placebo, arthritic symptoms significantly lessened whilst taking the Boswellia, but then returned with a vengeance when the treatment was switched over to placebo.[63] Other studies with arthritic patients have shown significant relief after four weeks supplementing 600mg of boswellic acid.[64]

Preparations are available in tablet and cream form – the ideal dose is 200–400mg, one to three times a day; the creams are especially useful in the treatment of localised inflammation.

◆ ASHWAGANDHA

Ashwagandha is a promising natural remedy that has been used for hundreds of years as part of the Ayurvedic medicine tradition in India. The active ingredients in this powerful natural anti-inflammatory herb are 'withanolides'. These also appear to have anti-cancer properties. In animal studies ashwagandha has proven highly effective against arthritis. In one study animals with arthritis were given either ashwagandha, hydrocortisone or placebo. While hydrocortisone produced a 44 per cent reduction in symptoms, ashwagandha produced an 89 per cent reduction in symptoms, making it substantially more effective than cortisone.[65]

Although this remedy has a good track record in Ayurvedic medicine it has only recently come to the attention of conventional medicine and human trials are awaited with interest. The therapeutic dose depends on the concentration of withanolides. Try 300mg twice a day of the root, providing 1.5 per cent withanolides.

◆ MSM

A naturally occurring organic form of sulphur, known as MSM, has been found to have remarkable health benefits, including better hair, nails and skin, and allergy relief. MSM (which stands for methylsulfonylmethane) is a source of the essential mineral sulphur which is one of the minerals most crucial to life. It is involved in a multitude of key body functions including pain control, inflammation, detoxification and tissue building.

A number of small trials have reported consistent relief from pain and inflammation in a variety of conditions, including back pain, joint pain and muscle pain.[66] MSM helps the body build and repair, as well as calming down inflammation. If you are prone to allergic or inflammatory health problems, such as eczema, asthma or hayfever, MSM may provide substantial relief.

MSM is available both as a balm and as capsules. For chronic pain, perhaps frequent headaches, back or muscle pain, try supplementing 1–3g a day. Start with 1g for a week, then double the dose. However, don't expect overnight results. It often takes a week or two to work and a few people have reported a flare-up of symptoms for a couple of days, as the sulphur helps the body detoxify and repair old injuries.

◆ GINGER

Ginger has been used for thousands of years in Eastern medicine. Whilst the learned doctors of this ancient and well-respected tradition knew that it was highly beneficial for reducing inflammation and rheumatism, they probably didn't know why. Twentieth-century technology has demonstrated that ginger inhibits the synthesis of pro-inflammatory prostaglandins and thromboxanes, another type of inflammatory mediator. It also has antioxidant properties and fresh ginger (not dried) contains an enzyme that may have a similar action to bromelain.[67]

In one study, supplementing ginger reduced pain and swelling in three-quarters of the participants with rheumatoid and osteoarthritis, while all patients with muscular discomfort experienced relief from pain.[68] Taking a supplement of 500–2000mg of ginger a day is ideal. Otherwise, incorporate a 1cm slice of fresh ginger into your daily diet.

◆ QUERCITIN

This is a potent antioxidant (see Chapter 6) which works with vitamins C and E to protect against free radical damage; it also has an anti-inflammatory effect because it inhibits the enzymes that produce pro-inflammatory prostaglandins.

Quercitin is a natural bioflavonoid that is increasingly featuring in the treatment of inflammatory diseases. Bioflavonoids frequently occur in nature alongside vitamin C. Quercitin is a non-citrus bioflavonoid found in onions, broccoli, squash and red grapes. It has been shown to inhibit the production of pro-inflammatory prostaglandins (type 2).[69] Quercitin also inhibits the release of histamine which is involved in inflammatory reactions, helps to stabilise cells, and reduces collagen breakdown and free radical activity, all of which are the markers of a good anti-inflammatory agent for arthritis. Quercitin is available in healthfood stores and is probably worth experimenting with in doses of 500mg a day, taken between meals.

Many plant foods contain such flavonoid compounds, which are known to inhibit inflammation.[70] These are found in fruits and vegetables and especially in red/blue foods such as berries and beetroot. This is one reason why vegetarian diets have proven highly effective in reducing pain and inflammation.

ANTI-INFLAMMATORY SUPPLEMENTS

This is one piece of the jigsaw that will make up your personal supplement programme (see page 138)

The easiest way to supplement these natural anti-inflammatory agents is in various combined herbal formulae. Since their effect is probably synergistic, this may prove more effective than just taking one ingredient alone. These remedies can also be found in the form of creams, used to reduce localised pain and swelling. An effective oral supplement might provide the following daily amounts, in addition to essential fats:

Curcumin	200–1500mg
Boswellia	200–1200mg
Ashwagandha	100–600mg
MSM	1–3g
Ginger	200–2000mg
Quercitin	100–1000mg

chapter 11

Bone-Building Nutrients

The ability to keep your bones strong (a prerequisite for preventing arthritis and osteoporosis) depends to a large extent on how your body makes use of calcium, magnesium and phosphorus. Of these, calcium is the most abundant mineral in bone. However, more and more evidence is accumulating to show that dietary calcium intake is only one of a number of factors that influence the proper use of calcium in the body.[71] The degeneration of cartilage seems to herald the beginning of osteoarthritis, the most common form of arthritis. And the cartilage of osteoarthritic sufferers appears to be different in composition from that of non-sufferers.[72]

WHAT IS CARTILAGE?

Cartilage is what we often call 'gristle' – the Adam's apple, the tip of the nose, bone ends, and the shock absorbers between our spinal vertebrae are all made of cartilage. It is a tough, elastic, translucent material. The cartilage at bone ends is called fibro-cartilage and is the strongest of all.

Cells that produce cartilage are called chondrocytes. Cartilage is made of collagen and proteoglycans (a complex of protein and carbohydrate) which together act as a kind of intercellular glue. It is this complex that is thought to give cartilage its special properties. Bone formation requires both the 'glue' (collagen and proteoglycans) and the bricks, which are principally calcium and phosphorus which combine into a compound known as hydroxyapatite.

HOW CAN CARTILAGE BE STRENGTHENED?

Much research has focused on ways of improving the body's ability to make healthy cartilage and heal joints. To this end, extracts from shark cartilage and green-lipped mussels have entered the repertoire of arthritis remedies. As bizarre as this may sound, there is a good reason for it. The green-lipped mussel contains high levels of protein, vitamins and minerals, and a type of proteoglycans, which is a natural joint lubricant and component of all cartilage. Shark cartilage, a recent addition to healthfood shop shelves, may have a similar effect. Most recently, though, glucosamine sulphate and chondroitin have become popular, effective and economical supplements for people with arthritis (see page xx).

The theory, in accordance with the basic principle of 'optimum nutrition', is that if you provide your body cells with the materials they need to do their job properly, they will. If arthritics lack the necessary components to make healthy cartilage, why not provide them? It is certainly far less invasive than giving drugs that suppress the symptoms but do nothing to stop the disease. Unlike other body tissue, cartilage has no blood or nerve supply. Cartilage relies on nutrients within the body's internal fluids which are moved around joint spaces by means of compression and relaxation. Thus, exercise is another way to improve nutrient transport to cartilage. During the day the cartilaginous discs between spinal vertebrae are compressed. At night, when we lie down, these discs expand, sucking in nutrients from surrounding body fluids.

◆ CALCIUM AND MAGNESIUM

Calcium is the most abundant mineral in the body, accounting for 1.6 per cent of our body mass. Of the 1200g of calcium in us, more than 99 per cent is in our bones and teeth. The rest is present in muscles, nerves and the bloodstream, where it plays a crucial role in many enzymes and the production of nerve signals and muscular energy.

Calcium is relatively well absorbed, with an average of 30 per cent of ingested calcium reaching the bloodstream. But its absorption into the bloodstream depends on many factors. An excess of alcohol, a lack of hydrochloric acid in the stomach, or an excess of acid-forming foods (mainly protein) decrease its absorption. So does the presence of lead, which competes with it for absorption sites.

Once in the body, there are many factors which influence calcium balance. Again, heavy metals like lead compete with calcium. So do sodium (salt), tea, cocoa and red wine. In post-menopausal women, the low levels of oestrogen also make calcium less retainable. One of the greatest factors in calcium balance is exercise or, rather, lack of it. Studies at NASA, where they discovered losses of calcium in astronauts in zero gravity, showed that weight-bearing exercise (for example, walking) could raise calcium levels in the body by 2 per cent or more.[73]

Once in the body, calcium is constantly moving from blood

to bone. It is released into the blood when it is needed to stimulate muscles or nerves. Once this reaction is over, the thyroid gland recalls calcium to the bones by secreting the hormone calcitonin. An imbalance in the thyroid or parathyroid gland can also interfere with calcium balance.

Bones contain magnesium and phosphorus, as well as calcium. While phosphorus is abundant in most people's diets, calcium and particularly magnesium are often lacking. Dairy produce, although a good source of calcium, is not a good source of magnesium. Nuts, seeds and root vegetables are good sources of both. Since most people's diet contains dairy produce, but little in the way of vegetables, nuts and seeds, magnesium deficiency is widespread. According to rough estimates, fewer than 20 per cent of people get enough magnesium.[74]

Without magnesium, calcium is unlikely to be used properly. Recent research has shown that magnesium-deficient infants cannot produce enough parathormone (PTH) to respond to low calcium levels in the blood, consequently resulting in calcium deficiency in the body.[75] What's more, the conversion of vitamin D into the active hormone that increases calcium retention is dependent on magnesium. In order to be incorporated into bone, calcium forms crystals, a process which is again facilitated by an enzyme that is magnesium-dependent.[76]

Low magnesium levels are associated with osteoporosis, and research by Dr Guy Abraham has shown remarkable results in reversing osteoporosis using a multi-nutrient approach including magnesium.[77] He studied 26 post-menopausal women all receiving hormone replacement therapy. All women were assessed for bone density. Seven patients received dietary advice similar to that recommended in this book, while 19 received the same dietary advice and six nutritional supplements. These provided a broad spectrum of vitamins and minerals, including 500mg of calcium and 600mg of magnesium.

At their return visits, 6 to 12 months later, bone density was measured again. Those with dietary advice and hormone replacement therapy had an insignificant 0.7 per cent increase in bone density, while those also taking supplements had a 16 times greater increase in bone density of 11 per cent. At the start of the study, 15 out of the 19 women due to take supplements had a bone density below the fracture threshold, indicating osteoporosis. Within a year of taking supplements only seven patients still had bone densities below this threshold. This study shows, without a doubt, how potent a combined intake of vitamins and minerals is for reversing bone disease, in comparison to standard drug treatment.

To ensure an adequate dietary intake of both these minerals, you should eat plenty of vegetables, especially green vegetables, for magnesium, and dairy produce, tinned sardines and soya products for calcium. Nuts, seeds and root vegetables are good sources of both. Do not, however, eat large amounts of dairy foods every day (i.e. with every meal), as this can actually cause you to lose calcium from the body.

♦ ZINC

Zinc is found in high concentrations in bone tissue and has an important role in bone formation. Research proves that zinc is important for those with osteoporosis or low bone density. In one study it was shown that there is a connection between low bone density and zinc deficiency in women with osteoporosis.[78]

Good sources of zinc are Brazil nuts, bean sprouts, oysters, peanuts, pecan nuts and pumpkin seeds. If supplementing zinc take the more absorbable forms which are zinc picolinate, glycinate and citrate. Take it separately from food and other supplements, especially calcium. (For more on zinc see Chapter 3.)

◆ BORON

Boron is an abundant trace element in soil, food and humans, although it has not yet been proven essential. It seems to have an important role in bone-building and strength; vitamin D and calcium both need boron to help them work properly. It can reduce loss of calcium because it locks calcium into the bone and it increases the proper activity of oestrogen (both very important for bone integrity). Research shows that boron is useful for improving low bone density as well as arthritis.

Dr Neilson and colleagues from the US Department of Agriculture investigated boron in relation to mineral and hormone balance in post-menopausal women.[79] They found that supplementing 3mg a day helped the body retain calcium and magnesium, especially in those with poor magnesium status. It also increased the levels of the hormones testosterone and oestradiol, related to oestrogen, which is the only agent so far tested that consistently increases bone density in post-menopausal women. According to Dr Neilson, 'The findings suggest that supplementation of a low-level diet with an amount of boron commonly found in diets high in fruit and vegetables induces changes in post-menopausal women consistent with the prevention of calcium loss and bone demineralisation.'

High levels of boron tend to be found in fruit such as

apples, pears, prunes, raisins, dates as well as honey, tomatoes and soya. Supplementation, up to 3mg a day, together with a high fruit and vegetable diet, would provide more than optimal intakes of this potentially important trace element.

♦ VITAMIN C

Vitamin C is vital for healthy joints. Both bone and cartilage formation depend on collagen as a building material; it is only synthesised in the presence of vitamin C. So a lack of vitamin C could quite possibly cause cartilage and bone abnormalities.

The optimum intake is likely to be anywhere between 1000mg and 10,000mg per day. If you drink excessive amounts of alcohol, live in a polluted city, have a stressful lifestyle, take drugs including aspirin, or smoke, your optimal intake will be raised. An intake of around 50mg per cigarette probably affords maximum protection. For anyone suffering from arthritis, 3–5g would be a sensible daily intake to assist healthy collagen formation of bone and cartilage. (For more on vitamin C see Chapter 2.)

♦ SILICA

Silicon is a trace mineral which is very important for skin, hair, ligaments and bone. It is needed for the formation of collagen in the bone and cartilage. There is some evidence to show that silica (the dioxide of silicone) is necessary to aid the formation of apatite crystal which is one of the main ingredients in our bones. In a study carried out by the Center Hospital of Toulon in 1993, women with osteoporosis were given silicon, fluoride, magnesium and etidrodonate to see if they made a difference to bone density. One year later it was found that the women who had received silicon supplementation had a significant increase in their bone density.[80]

Silica is found mainly in fresh vegetables, especially cabbage, lettuce, parsnips, asparagus, olives and radishes, and also in wholegrains. Unfortunately, modern food processing strips away the silica content of many foods, especially cereals and wholegrains. Therefore it is very important to ensure that you eat plenty of fresh vegetables and unprocessed wholegrains.

You can find silica in most of the combined bone-building supplements. The most commonly used source is the herb horsetail. If you have low bone density or osteoporosis, you should take 25–50mg each day.

◆ VITAMIN D AND VITAMIN K

Vitamin D is needed to help the body use calcium properly. It is converted into a hormone, calcitriol, that works with parathormone to promote the absorption and retention of calcium. Vitamin D deficiency among the elderly is far from uncommon. According to a survey published in the *New England Journal of Medicine*, 57 per cent of 290 senior citizens in hospital had low blood levels of this bone-building vitamin.[81]

Vitamin D can be made in the skin in the presence of sunlight, which may be one reason why arthritis sufferers often feel better in the summer. It is also present in meat, fish, eggs and milk. Some meat-eaters get too much vitamin D from eating these foods, plus foods fortified with vitamin D. However, if you don't eat these foods often it is best to supplement 400iu of vitamin D each day.

In summary, the body can use calcium better (helping to

make strong bones, joints and healthy cartilage) if your diet also provides adequate amounts of magnesium and vitamin D. Supplementing an extra 500mg of calcium and magnesium, plus 400iu of vitamin D is likely to offer optimal protection for bones and joints.

Vitamin K, previously only thought to play a role in blood clotting, may also be important for healthy bones. Bone contains significant amounts of vitamin K. Low blood levels are found in those with osteoporosis and in post-menopausal women and this has led to speculation that vitamin K supplementation may help to maintain and improve bone density. There is some evidence that supplementation can speed up recovery from osteoporosis. (See Chapter 2.)

◆ GLUCOSAMINE SULPHATE AND CHONDROITIN

Glucosamine sulphate (GS) is an essential part of cell membranes and the cellular 'glue'. It therefore plays a fundamental role in the formation of joints, tendons, ligaments, synovial fluid, bone and many more body parts including skin and blood vessels. Cartilage in joints consists of cells embedded in collagen that sits within a framework of watery 'proteoglycan' gel – it is the integrity of this structure that allows for the flexibility of joints and their ability to resist the pressure of impact and gravity. The building blocks for this proteoglycan comes from GS which some people seem less able to make as they get older.

GS appears to stop or reverse joint degeneration by directly providing the body with the materials needed for the formation of the proteoglycans – the framework for joint structure; it may also prevent the breakdown of this substance in the body.[82] Joint cartilage contains a higher concentration of GS than any other structural tissue.[83] Chondroitin also helps the formation of proteoglycans.

Several experiments have shown GS and chondroitin to be effective in alleviating arthritis. In one such study pain was reduced in as many as 80 per cent of volunteers who had degeneration in the knee, while inflammation was reduced in two-thirds of them.[84] The scientists reported that GS appeared to produce better results overall, especially in the people with mild arthritis, although chondroitin was more successful in advanced cases.

The usual dosage for GS is 500mg, three times daily; many people find the longer they use it, the more beneficial it feels.

 10 BONE-BUILDING SUPPLEMENTS

This is one piece of the jigsaw that will make up your personal supplement programme (see page 138)

In summary, a good bone-building supplement might contain the following nutrients:

Calcium	300–500mg
Magnesium	200–300mg
Zinc	8–15mg
Boron	1–3mg
Vitamin C	100–300mg
Silica	25–50mg
Vitamin D	2.5–5µg (100–200iu)
Vitamin K	50–200mcg
Glucosamine	500–1500mg (usually a separate supplement)
Chondroitin	500–1500mg

part 3

chapter 12

Everything You Need to Know About Supplements

V itamin supplements can be enormously beneficial in
helping our bodies cope with a stressful twentieth-
century lifestyle. But not all supplements are the same.
Depending on which multivitamin tablet you choose, getting
the basic optimum vitamin requirements can cost you
anywhere between 30p (20c) and over £5 ($7.50) a day! And,
with so many supplements available, all promising perfect
health, it's easy to get confused. For instance, if you're looking
for a simple multivitamin preparation to meet the basic
optimum requirements, you have at least 20 products to
choose from. So picking the right supplements is an art in
itself! This chapter explains what to look for in a good supplement.

◆ READING THE LABEL

Labelling laws vary from country to country, but most of the
principles are the same. Depending on the ingredients, different laws apply and, since these change from time to time,

many manufacturers are almost as confused as members of the public. Figure 10 shows a typical product. Here's how to read the small print.

This will give you some idea of what to look out for – the dosages are correct, the chemical names for the different vitamins are given, and the filler (calcium phosphate) is listed. Directions for when and how to take the tablets are given, as well as extra information and a guarantee of quality. These are the things to look for when you are buying supplements: do not be misled by an attractive-looking label or a very cheap price, but do not pay too much either. Unfortunately, not all supplements are true to their labels – reputable vitamin companies should give you a list of all the ingredients.

VITAMIN NAMES AND THEIR AMOUNTS

For most supplements, the ingredients have to be listed in order of weight, starting with the one present in the greatest quantity. This is often confusing since the non-nutrient additives needed to make the tablet are included in this list. In the case of calcium phosphate, which is used as a 'filler', it does also provide nutritional benefit, so it is a good filler substance to use. Often the chemical name of the nutrient is used instead of the common vitamin code (for example, ergocalciferol for vitamin D). These names are listed below.

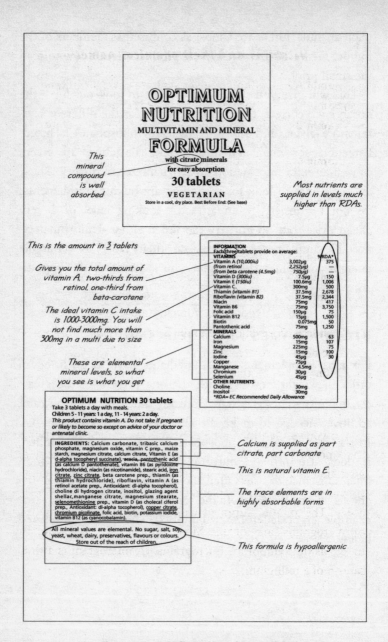

OPTIMUM NUTRITION
MULTIVITAMIN AND MINERAL
FORMULA

with citrate minerals
for easy absorption

30 tablets

VEGETARIAN

Store in a cool, dry place. Best Before End: (See base)

This mineral compound is well absorbed

Most nutrients are supplied in levels much higher than RDAs.

This is the amount in 3 tablets

Gives you the total amount of vitamin A, two-thirds from retinol, one-third from beta-carotene

The ideal vitamin C intake is 1000-3000mg. You will not find much more than 300mg in a multi due to size

These are 'elemental' mineral levels, so what you see is what you get

INFORMATION
Each (three) tablets provide on average:

VITAMINS		*RDA*
Vitamin A (10,000iu)	3,002µg	375
(from retinol	2,252µg)	—
(from beta carotene (4.5mg)	750µg)	—
Vitamin D (300iu)	7.5µg	150
Vitamin E (150iu)	100.6mg	1,006
Vitamin C	300mg	500
Thiamin (vitamin B1)	37.5mg	2,678
Riboflavin (vitamin B2)	37.5mg	2,344
Niacin	75mg	417
Vitamin B6	75mg	3,750
Folic acid	150µg	75
Vitamin B12	15µg	1,500
Biotin	0.075mg	50
Pantothenic acid	75mg	1,250
MINERALS		
Calcium	500mg	63
Iron	15mg	107
Magnesium	225mg	75
Zinc	15mg	100
Iodine	45µg	30
Copper	75µg	
Manganese	4.5mg	
Chromium	30µg	
Selenium	45µg	
OTHER NUTRIENTS		
Choline	30mg	
Inositol	30mg	

*RDA= EC Recommended Daily Allowance

OPTIMUM NUTRITION 30 tablets
Take 3 tablets a day with meals.
Children 5 - 11 years: 1 a day, 11 - 14 years: 2 a day.
This product contains vitamin A. Do not take if pregnant or likely to become so except on advice of your doctor or antenatal clinic.

INGREDIENTS: Calcium carbonate, tribasic calcium phosphate, magnesium oxide, vitamin C prep., maize starch, magnesium citrate, calcium citrate, Vitamin E (as d-alpha tocopheryl succinate), acacia, pantothenic acid (as calcium D pantothenate), vitamin B6 (as pyridoxine hydrochloride), niacin (as nicotinamide), stearic acid, iron citrate, zinc citrate, beta carotene prep., thiamin (as thiamin hydrochloride), riboflavin, vitamin A (as retinol acetate prep.), Antioxidant: dl-alpha tocopherol), choline di hydrogen citrate, inositol, glazing agent shellac, manganese citrate, magnesium stearate, selenomethionine prep., vitamin D (as cholecal ciferol prep., Antioxidant: dl-alpha tocopherol), copper citrate, chromium picolinate, folic acid, biotin, potassium iodide, vitamin B12 (as cyanocobalamin).

All mineral values are elemental. No sugar, salt, soy, yeast, wheat, dairy, preservatives, flavours or colours. Store out of the reach of children.

Calcium is supplied as part citrate, part carbonate

This is natural vitamin E.

The trace elements are in highly absorbable forms

This formula is hypoallergenic

Figure 10 – Reading a supplement label

Vitamins and their chemical names

Vitamin A – retinol, retinyl palmitate or beta-carotene

Vitamin D – ergocalciferol or cholecalciferol

Vitamin E – d(l) alpha tocopherol, tocopheryl acetate or tocopheryl succinate

Vitamin C – ascorbic acid or calcium/magnesium/sodium ascorbate

Vitamin B1 – thiamine, thiamine hydrochloride, thiamine mononitrate

Vitamin B2 – riboflavin

Vitamin B3 – niacin, niacinamide

Vitamin B5 – pantothenic acid, calcium pantothenate

Vitamin B6 – pyridoxine, pyridoxal-5-phosphate, pyridoxine hydrochloride

Vitamin B12 – cyanocobalamin

Folic acid – folate

Biotin – biotin

When you've identified which nutrient is which, then look at the amount provided by each daily dose. Some supplements give the amount in two tablets, stating 'Each two tablets provide ...' since the supplement is designed to be taken twice a day. The amount supplied will be given in milligrams (mg) or micrograms (mcg or µg). Most countries are now switching to 'µg' as the symbol for micrograms. (A microgram is a thousandth of a milligram.)

ELEMENTAL MINERALS

Minerals in multivitamin and mineral tablets often omit the 'elemental' value of the compound, stating only the amount of the mineral compound. For instance, 100mg of zinc amino acid chelate will provide only 10mg of zinc and 90mg of the amino acid to which it is chelated (attached).

You want to know the amount of the actual mineral – in this example, 10mg. This is called the 'elemental value'. Most reputable manufacturers make your life easy by stating something like 'zinc amino acid chelate (providing 5mg zinc) 50mg' or 'zinc (as amino acid chelate) 5mg', both of which mean you are getting 5mg of elemental, or actual zinc. Otherwise, you may have to contact the manufacturer for more detailed information. Most good companies declare this information either on the label or in literature that comes with the product.

Supplement labels are also required to show the percentage of the RDA that is met by the product. For the purposes of achieving optimum nutrition, this is largely irrelevant, since the amounts needed for optimal health are often many times higher than the RDA, so you will find figures like '860% of RDA'.

FILLERS, BINDERS, LUBRICANTS AND COATINGS

Supplements often contain other ingredients necessary for their production. While capsules don't really need anything added, tablets usually do in order to allow the ingredients to stick together. Tablets start off as powders. To get the bulk right, 'fillers' are added. 'Binders' are added to give the mixture the right consistency and lubricants are also used. Only when this is done can the mixture be turned into small, uneven granules, which are then pressed into tablets under considerable force. Granulating allows the mixture to lock together, forming a solid mass. The tablet may then be covered with a 'protein coating' to protect it from deterioration and make it easier to swallow.

Unfortunately, many tablets also have artificial colouring and flavouring added, as well as a sugar coating. For instance, many vitamin C tablets are made to look orange and taste sweet, since we associate vitamin C with oranges! Vitamin C is naturally almost white and certainly isn't sweet – and nor should your supplement be. As a rule of thumb, only buy supplements that declare their fillers and binders (sometimes also called 'excipients'). Companies with integrity are usually only too happy to display this information. The following fillers and binders are fine to use and some add extra nutritious properties to the tablet.

Dicalcium phosphate – a natural filler providing calcium and phosphate

Cellulose – a natural binder consisting of plant fibre

Alginic acid/sodium alginate – a natural binder from seaweed

Gum acacia/gum arabic – a natural vegetable gum

Calcium or magnesium stearate – a natural lubricant (usually from an animal source)

Silica – a natural lubricant

Zein – a corn protein for coating the tablet

Brazil wax – a natural coating, from palm trees

Stearate, which is the chemical name for saturated fat, is used as a lubricant. The cheapest variety is animal source, although non-animal source stearates are available. If you're a strict vegetarian you may want to check this with the supplement company. If a product is labelled 'suitable for vegans' it cannot legally contain any animal source ingredients.

Most large tablets are coated. This makes them shiny, smooth and easier to swallow. This isn't so necessary with small tablets. If a tablet is 'chalky' or rough on the outside then it isn't coated. Coating, depending on the substance used, can also protect the ingredients, increasing their shelf-life. Avoid sugar-coated, artificially coloured supplements. Natural colours, from berry extracts for example, are fine.

Occasionally, a manufacturer over-coats a batch of tablets and, particularly for those with poor digestion or a lack of stomach acid, this can inhibit the tablet's disintegration. Most reliable companies check the disintegration time on each batch to rule out this possibility.

FREE FROM SUGAR, GLUTEN, ETC ...

Many of the better supplements will also declare that the product is free from sugar and gluten. If you are allergic to milk or yeast do check that the tablets are also free from lactose (milk sugar) and yeast. B vitamins can be derived from yeast, so you need to be careful. If in doubt, contact the company and ask for an independent 'assay' of the ingredients – good companies will supply this information. Sometimes glucose, fructose or dextrose is used to sweeten a tablet and yet the tablet still declares 'no sugar'. These are best avoided. A small amount of fructose is the least evil if you're having diffi-culty enticing a child to take vitamins. Any other preservatives or flavouring agents should be avoided unless they are natural. For instance, pineapple essence is a natural additive.

If you are vegan or vegetarian choose supplements that state this. Retinol (vitamin A) can either be derived from animal source, artificially made or derived from a vegetable source, such as retinyl palmitate. Vitamin D can be artificially made, derived from sheep wool or from a vegetable source. Companies are not legally required to state the source of the nutrients, just their chemical form.

◆ BUILDING YOUR OWN SUPPLEMENT PROGRAMME

Now you know how to read the labels and find out if a particular supplement contains what you need, here's how to turn your nutrient needs into a supplement programme.

Theoretically, you could take a mega-mega-multi that has everything you could possibly need in it. The trouble is, this would be enormous, impossible to swallow and no doubt give you a lot more than you need of some nutrients. The other extreme is to take one supplement for each vitamin, exactly matching your requirements – but you'd end up with handfuls of pills.

Instead, nutritionists use 'formulae' – combinations of nutrients – that, when combined appropriately, more or less reach your needs. In a typical supplement programme you may end up with four supplements to take. These formulae are like building blocks. The essential building blocks are shown in Figure 11.

VITAMIN C

It is worth taking vitamin C separately because the amount you need won't fit in a multi. The supplement should provide around 1000mg of vitamin C. Some vitamin C formulae also

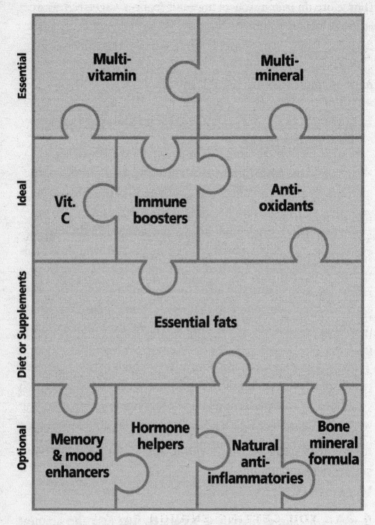

Figure 11 – Building your supplement programme

provide other key immune-boosting nutrients such as bioflavonoids or anthocyanidins, zinc, cat's claw, or echinacea. (For more on immune-boosing nutrients see Chapter 7.)

2 MULTIVITAMIN

A good multivitamin should contain at least 7500iu of A, 400iu of D, 100iu of E, 250mg of C and 50mg of B1, B2, B3, B5 and B6, 10mcg of B12, 50mcg of folic acid and biotin.

3 MULTIMINERAL

This should provide at least 150mg of calcium, 75mg of magnesium, 10mg of iron, 10mg of zinc, 2.5mg of manganese, 20mcg of chromium and 25mcg of selenium, and, ideally, some molybdenum, vanadium and boron.

Don't be tempted by a multivitamin and mineral. You simply can't fit all of the above vitamins and minerals into one tablet. Good, combined multivitamin and mineral formulae therefore recommend two or more tablets a day to meet these kinds of levels. The bulkiest nutrients are vitamin C, calcium and magnesium. These are often insufficiently supplied in multivitamin and mineral formulae. With the exception of vitamin C, which is best taken separately, a good multivitamin and mineral formula should meet all the '0 to 4' nutrient levels in Figure 4 (page 25), providing the foundation for your supplement programme.

4 ARE YOU GETTING ENOUGH FAT?

There are two ways of meeting your essential fat requirements. One is from diet, either by eating a heaped tablespoon of ground seeds every day, having a tablespoon of special cold-pressed seed oils and/or eating fish three times a week. The other is to supplement concentrated oils. For Omega 3 this means either flax seed oil capsules or the more concentrated fish oil capsules providing EPA and DHA. For Omega 6 this means supplementing a source of GLA such as evening primrose oil or borage oil. For certain conditions, such as PMS or arthritis, it is helpful to do both. (For more on essential fats see Chapter 4.)

5 ADD EXTRA ANTIOXIDANT NUTRIENTS

The evidence is now very conclusive that an optimal intake of antioxidant nutrients slows down the ageing process and prevents a variety of diseases. For this reason it is well worth supplementing extra antioxidant nutrients – on top of those in a good multivitamin – to ensure that you are achieving the best possible anti-ageing protection. The kind of nutrients that are provided in an antioxidant supplement are vitamins A, C, E and beta-carotene, zinc and selenium, possibly iron, copper and manganese, the amino acids glutathione or cysteine, plus antioxidants like bilberry extract, pycnogenol, grape seed extract, etc. These plant antioxidants, rich in bioflavonoids and anthocyanidins, are also often supplied in more comprehensive vitamin C formulae. (For more on antioxidants see Chapter 6.)

6 IMMUNE-BOOSTING NUTRIENTS

Key immune-boosting nutrients such as bioflavonoids or anthocyanidins, zinc, cat's claw or echinacea can be found in some vitamin C formulae. (For more on immune-boosting nutrients see Chapter 7.)

OPTIONAL EXTRAS

Depending on your needs, you may wish to supplement various optional extras. These include:

7 Memory and mood-enhancing nutrients (for more on these see Chapter 8)

8 Hormone helpers (for more on these see Chapter 9)

9 Natural pain-killers and anti-inflammatories (for more on these see Chapter 10)

10 Bone-building nutrients (for more on these see Chapter 11).

INDIVIDUAL NUTRIENTS

Sometimes even the above formulas may still leave you short on specific nutrients if you have particularly high needs, based on the Nutrient Check on page 16. Common shortfalls are vitamin B3 (niacin), vitamin B5 (pantothenate), vitamin B6 (pyridoxine), and chromium. If you need both vitamin B3 and chromium, take chromium polynicotinate which is a complex of B3 and chromium. If you need extra B3 be aware that niacin makes you blush. Niacinamide or 'no-flush niacin' does not. You may prefer these forms although there is nothing wrong with blushing.

A Directory of Recommended Supplement Companies whose products meet these recommended levels of vitamin and mineral intake is given on page 181.

◆ WHEN TO TAKE YOUR SUPPLEMENTS

Now that you've worked out what to take, you'll want to know when to take them. This depends not only on what is technically best, but also on your lifestyle. If taking supplements twice a day would mean that you'd forget the second lot, you're probably better off taking them all at once. After all, nature supplies them all in one go, with a meal. Here are the 'ten commandments' of supplement-taking:

1. Take vitamins and minerals a few minutes before or after or during a meal.

2. Take most of your supplements with your first meal of the day.

3. Don't take B vitamins late at night if you have difficulty sleeping.

4. Take extra minerals, especially calcium and magnesium, in the evening – these help you sleep.

5. If you're taking two or more B complex or vitamin C tablets, take one at each meal.

6. Don't take individual B vitamins unless you are also taking a general B complex, perhaps in a multivitamin.

7. Don't take individual minerals unless you are also taking a general multimineral.

8. If you are anaemic (iron-deficient) take extra iron with vitamin C.

9. Always take at least ten times as much zinc as copper. If you know you are copper-deficient take copper only with ten times as much zinc, e.g. 0.5mg copper to 5mg zinc.

10. Take your supplements every day – irregular supplementation doesn't work.

On a practical note, I have found that one of two supplement-taking strategies works for most people. Either take most in the morning, and a few in the evening so you don't have to take any to work. Or, if your supplement programme consists of, say, three multis, three vitamin Cs and three antioxidants, put all three in one jar or an old camera film container and take one of each with each meal. Always keep a small container in your handbag or briefcase so they're on hand when you eat.

◆ ARE THERE ANY SIDE-EFFECTS?

The only side-effects of optimum nutrition are increased energy, mental alertness and a greater resistance to disease. In fact, a survey of supplement-takers found that 79 per cent noticed a definite improvement in energy, 66 per cent felt more emotionally balanced, 60 per cent had better memory and mental alertness, skin condition improved in 55 per cent of people, and 61 per cent had noticed a definite improvement in their overall well-being. As long as you stick to the levels given in this book and don't take toxic levels the only side-effects are beneficial ones.

A small number of people do, however, experience slight symptoms on starting a supplement programme. This may be because they take too many supplements with too little food, or perhaps because a supplement contains something that doesn't agree with them, such as yeast. These problems are usually solved by stopping the supplements, then taking one only for four days, then adding another for the next four days, and so on until all supplements are taken. This procedure will usually tell you if there is a supplement that is causing a problem. More often than not, the problem simply goes away.

Sometimes people feel worse before they feel better. This is because the body has got used to coping with the onslaught of pollution, poor diet, toxins and stimulants. Then it suddenly gets a wonderful diet and all the supplements it needs. This can lead to 'detoxification' – the body cleansing itself – which is not a bad thing and usually subsides within a month. However, if you have inexplicable symptoms on starting a supplement programme or are suffering in any way, see a clinical nutritionist.

◆ WHAT HEALTH IMPROVEMENTS CAN I EXPECT?

Vitamins and minerals are not drugs, so you shouldn't expect an overnight improvement in your health. Most people experience definite improvement within three months. This is the shortest length of time that you should experiment with a supplement programme. The earliest noticeable health changes are increased energy, mental alertness, emotional stability and improvements in the condition of the skin – these are usually experienced within a month. Your health will continue to improve as long as you are following the right programme. My health is still improving after 20 years! If you do not experience any noticeable improvement in three months, it is best to see a clinical nutritionist.

◆ HOW OFTEN SHOULD I REASSESS MY NEEDS?

When you first start taking supplements your needs will change, so a reassessment every three months is sensible. Your nutrient needs should decrease as you get healthier.

Remember, you need optimum nutrition most when you are stressed. So when emergencies occur, or when you're working especially hard, make doubly sure that you eat well and take your supplements every day.

chapter 13

Choosing the Best Supplements

W hile the golden rule of any supplement programme is to take the right doses and take them regularly, there are many other issues to consider when choosing supplements. For instance, is it better to have natural rather than synthetic nutrients? Are capsules better than tablets? Are certain forms of minerals better absorbed? Are there good and bad combinations? What if you're on medication? Are there any drug–nutrient interactions or situations when you shouldn't take supplements?

◆ CAPSULES VERSUS TABLETS

Capsules used to be made of gelatin, which is an animal product and therefore not suitable for vegetarians. However, thanks to technological advances, capsules made from vegetable cellulose are now available. These are not yet available for 'softgel' capsules used for oils like vitamin E. The advantage of tablets is that, through compression, you can get more nutrients into them. The disadvantage is the need for fillers and binders. Some people think capsules allow better nutrient absorption, but, provided the tablet is properly made, there is little difference. Most vitamins can be provided as tablets, including the oil-based vitamins. For instance, natural vitamin E comes in two forms: d-alpha tocopherol acetate (oil); or d-alpha tocopherol succinate (powder). Both are equally potent.

◆ NATURAL VERSUS SYNTHETIC

A great deal of nonsense has been written about the advantages of natural vitamins. First of all, many products claiming to be natural simply aren't. By law, a certain percentage of a product must be natural for the product to be declared 'natural'. The percentage varies from country to country. By means of careful wording on the labels, some supplements sound natural but really aren't. For instance, 'vitamin C with rosehips' invariably means synthetic vitamin C with added rosehips, although it is often confused with vitamin C from rosehips. So which is better?

By definition, a synthetic vitamin must contain all the properties of the vitamin found in nature. If it doesn't, then the chemists haven't done their job properly. This is the case with vitamin E: natural d-alpha tocopherol succinate is 36 per cent more potent than the synthetic vitamin E called dl-alpha tocopherol (in this case the 'l' dictates the chemical difference). So natural vitamin E, usually derived from wheatgerm or soya oil, is better.

However, synthetic vitamin C (ascorbic acid) has the same biological potency as the natural substance, according to Dr Linus Pauling. No one has yet shown that natural vitamin C is more potent or beneficial to take. Indeed, most vitamin C is synthesised by taking a 'natural' sugar, such as dextrose, and two chemical reactions later you have ascorbic acid. This is little different from the chemical reactions that take place in animals that convert sugar to vitamin C. Vitamin C derived from, say, acerola cherries – the most concentrated source – is also considerably bulkier and more expensive. Acerola is only 20 per cent vitamin C, so a 1000mg tablet would be five times as large as a normal tablet and would cost you ten times as much!

It is true that vitamins derived from natural sources may contain unknown elements that increase their potency. Vitamin E – d-alpha tocopherol – is found with other toco-pherols (beta, gamma and delta tocopherol) in nature, so the inclusion of these with a measured amount of d-alpha toco-pherol may be of benefit. Vitamin C is found in nature together with the bioflavonoids – active nutrients that appear to increase its potency, particularly in its role of strengthening the capillaries (tiny blood vessels). Good sources of bioflavonoids are berries and citrus fruit, so the addition of citrus bioflavonoids or berry extracts to vitamin C tablets is one step closer to nature.

It is possible that yeast and rice bran, which are excellent sources of B vitamins, also contain unknown beneficial ingre-dients, so these vitamins are best supplied with yeast or rice bran. Brewer's yeast tablets or powder are far less efficient ways of taking B vitamins than B complex vitamin supple-ments with a little added yeast – one would have to eat pounds of yeast tablets to get optimum levels of B vitamins. However, watch out for yeast – some people are allergic to it, so if you react badly to any vitamin supplements, it could be yeast that is causing the problem. For this reason many supplements are yeast-free.

There are many other potentially helpful substances that may be provided with nutrients in a complex. Included here are co-enzymes that help to convert the nutrient into its active form. Vitamin B6, for example, needs to be converted from pyridoxine to pyridoxal-5-phosphate before it becomes active in the body. For this reason a number of B6 supplements contain zinc which helps this process. There are now supplements of pyridoxal-5-phosphate which should, theoretically, be more usable. Time will tell how much of an advantage such innovations will prove to be. But the key point is to make sure you get enough of each of the essential nutrients.

◆ VITAMIN AND MINERAL ABSORPTION

Vitamins and particularly minerals come in different forms which affect their absorption and availability. Apart from the form of the nutrient, there are also dietary and lifestyle factors that can help or hinder their bioavailability. Figure 13 shows you which forms of vitamins and minerals are best absorbed, and the factors that affect their absorption.

WATER-SOLUBLE NUTRIENTS

Vitamin or mineral	Best form	When best to take	What helps absorption	What hinders absorption
B1	thiamine	alone or with meals	B complex manganese	alcohol, stress, antibiotics
B2	riboflavin	alone or with meals	B complex	alcohol, tobacco, stress, antibiotics
B3	nicotinic acid, nicotinamide	alone or with meals	B complex	alcohol, stress, antibiotics
B5	calcium pantothenate	alone or with meals	biotin, folic acid, B complex	antibiotics, stress
B6	pyridoxine hydrochloride phosphate	alone or with meals	zinc, magnesium B complex	alcohol antibiotics, stress

Figure 12 – Maximising absorption of vitamins and minerals

Vitamin or mineral	Best form	When best to take	What helps absorption	What hinders absorption
B12	cyanocobalamin	alone or with meals	calcium, B complex	alcohol, intestinal parasites, stress, antibiotics
C	ascorbic acid, calcium ascorbate	away from meals	hydrochloric acid in stomach	heavy meals
Folic Acid		alone or with meals	C, B complex	alcohol, stress antibiotics
Biotin		alone or with meals	B complex	avidin (in raw egg whites), stress, antibiotics

FAT SOLUBLE VITAMINS

A	retinol, beta-carotene	take with foods containing fats or oils	zinc, E, C	lack of bile
E	D-alpha tocopherol	take with foods containing fats or oils	selenium, C	lack of bile, ferric forms of iron, oxidised fats
D	ergocalciferol, cholecalciferol	take with foods containing fats or oils	calcium, phosphorous E, C	lack of bile

MINERALS

Calcium – Ca	with protein food	magnesium, D, hydrochloric acid in stomach	Tea, coffee, smoking	
Magnesium – Mg	with protein food	calcium, B6, D, hydrochloric acid in stomach	Alcohol, tea, coffee, smoking	
Iron – Fe	with food	C, hydrochloric acid in stomach	oxalic acid, tea, coffee, smoking	
Zinc – Zn	on an empty stomach, p.m.	B6, C, hydrochloric acid in stomach	phytic acid, lead, copper, calcium, tea, coffee	
Manganese – Mn	with protein food	C, hydrochloric acid in stomach	high dosage zinc, tea, coffee, smoking	
Selenium – Se	on an empty stomach	E, hydrochloric acid in stomach	coffee, mercury tea, coffee,	
Chromium – Cr	with protein food	B3, hydrochloric acid in stomach	tea, coffee, smoking	

MINERAL BIOAVAILABILITY

Most of the minerals essential for health are supplied from food to the body as a compound, bound to a larger (food) molecule. This binding is known as chelation, from the Greek word *chela*, meaning 'a claw'. Some form of chelation is important, since most essential minerals in their 'raw' state are positively charged. The gut wall is negatively charged, so once separated from food through the process of digestion, these unbound positively charged minerals would be attracted to the gut wall. Instead of being absorbed, they would then easily become bound to undesirable substances like phytic acid in bran, tannic acid in tea, oxalic acid in spinach and so on. Once bound to the acids, the minerals would pass straight through the body.

The bioavailability of a mineral (i.e. the proportion of a nutrient that can be utilised by the body) depends on many factors, including the amount of 'enhancers' and 'inhibitors' present, such as phytates, other minerals and vitamins, and the acidity of the digestive environment. Most minerals are absorbed in the duodenum (the first part of the small intestine), assisted by the presence of stomach acid.

Minerals are bound, or chelated, to different compounds to help their absorption. Amino acid chelated minerals are bound to amino acids, examples of which are chromium picolinate, selenocysteine or zinc amino acid chelate. These are well absorbed, as are other 'organic' compounds such as citrates, gluconates and aspartates. Inorganic compounds, such as carbonates, sulphates and oxides, are less well absorbed.

For some minerals the extra cost of amino acid chelated minerals outweighs the advantage. For example, magnesium amino acid chelate is only twice as well absorbed as magne-

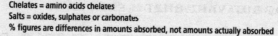

Chelates = amino acids chelates
Salts = oxides, sulphates or carbonates
% figures are differences in amounts absorbed, not amounts actually absorbed

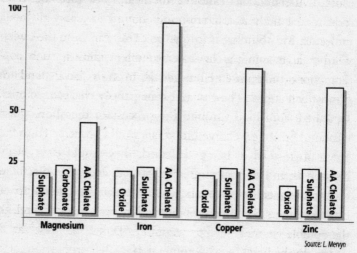

Source: L. Mervyn

Figure 13 – Comparison of bioavailability of mineral compounds

sium carbonate, an inexpensive source of magnesium. Iron amino acid chelate, on the other hand, is four times better absorbed, making the price differential worth it. Generally speaking, the following forms are most available to the body, listed in order of their bioavailability.

Calcium and magnesium – amino acid chelate, citrate, gluconate, carbonate

Iron – amino acid chelate, gluconate, sulphate, oxide

Zinc – picolinate, amino acid chelate, citrate, gluconate, sulphate

Chromium – picolinate, polynicotinate, gluconate

Selenium – selenocysteine or selenomethionine, sodium selenite

Manganese – amino acid chelate, citrate, gluconate

WHAT ABOUT SUSTAINED RELEASE?

Some vitamins are called prolonged, sustained or time-released, implying that the ingredients are not all made available for absorption in one go. This can be useful when taking large amounts of water-soluble vitamins, such as B complex or vitamin C. However, absorption also depends on the person and on the dosage. Some people are able to absorb and use 1000mg of vitamin C taken in one dose, so taking it in sustained release form would provide little benefit. However, if you take three 1000mg tablets each day, sustained release would allow you to take them all in one go. Since sustained-release vitamins are more expensive, one has to weigh up the pros and cons. There is no point in having a sustained-release fat-soluble vitamin, such as vitamin A, D or E, as these can be stored in the body.

The best sustained-release products are capsules containing tiny 'beads', each containing the desired nutrients, which dissolve at different rates, thus releasing the nutrients over time. This method, however, takes up a lot of space, so the dose isn't usually very high, which reduces the need for sustained release.

◆ GOOD AND BAD COMBINATIONS

The general rule is to take supplements with food. This is primarily because the presence of stomach acid enhances the absorption of many minerals, and the fat-soluble vitamins are carried by fats or oils which are present in most meals. Nutrients do, however, compete for absorption. For example, if a person wants to absorb a large amount of a specific amino acid such as lysine (good for preventing herpes), more will be absorbed if it is taken on an empty stomach or with non-protein food such as a piece of fruit. Similarly, a tiny mineral like selenium will be absorbed better on its own than as part of a multimineral.

However, no one wants to end up taking each supplement separately, so, unless you have a specific need or deficiency and want to maximise absorption by taking the nutrient on its own, it's best to spread your nutrients out through the day and take them with meals, as nature intended.

The exception that proves the rule is if you want to take the alkaline-forming 'ascorbate' type of vitamin C in quite large doses (3g or more a day). In this case, you should take it separately from meals to avoid neutralising stomach acidity. If you ever experience a burning sensation after taking vitamin C as ascorbic acid (a weak acid), one possibility is that you have some gastro-intestinal irritation or even an ulcer. See your doctor and have this checked out. While vitamin C helps to heal wounds, the acid form can irritate an existing problem and should be avoided.

◆ DRUG–NUTRIENT INTERACTIONS

There are very few dangerous drug–nutrient interactions, but there are many drugs which interfere with the action of nutrients, thereby increasing your need:

- **Aspirin** increases the need for vitamin C

- **The birth control pill** and **HRT** increase the need for B6, B12, folic acid and zinc

- **Antibiotics** increase the need for B vitamins and beneficial bacteria

- **Paracetamol** increases the need for antioxidants

Potentially dangerous combinations are:

- **Warfarin (a blood-thinning drug), aspirin, vitamin E and high EPA/DHA fish oils:** These all thin the blood and the combined effect is likely to be too strong. It is better to reduce the drugs and increase the nutrients, but first check with your doctor.

- **MAOI anti-depressants (such as Nardil or Parstelin) and yeast-containing supplements:** Yeast and alcohol and specific foods must be avoided while on these drugs.

- **Anti-convulsants and folic acid:** Some anti-convulsant drugs are anti-folate, creating an increased need, yet supplementation can impair the action of the drug. Specialist advice from your doctor and clinical nutritionist is recommended. For epileptics, be careful of supplementing the brain nutrient DMAE or high-dose essential fatty acids such as evening primrose oil.

- **Folic acid without B12:** In cases of B12 deficiency, supplementing folic acid can reduce symptoms while the underlying deficiency gets worse. Therefore, it is best to supplement both nutrients, preferably as part of a B complex.

◆ DOS AND DON'TS OF SUPPLEMENT TAKING

Very few problems occur with vitamin supplements. However, it is good to be aware of the following:

- **Vitamin A** (retinol) in doses in excess of 10,000iu (3000mcg) should not be given to pregnant women or women trying to conceive.

- **Beta-carotene**, in excess, makes your skin go yellow. If you have excessively yellowing skin check your beta-carotene intake from food and supplements. (This is quite different from jaundice or hepatitis in which the eyes go yellow too.)

- **Vitamin B2** (riboflavin) makes your urine bright yellow. This is normal.

- **Vitamin B3** in the form of niacin, usually in doses of 100mg or more, can make you flush, and go red, hot and itchy for up to 30 minutes. This is normal and is not an allergy. While beneficial, if you do not like it you can take less or take half the dose twice a day. Your flushing potential decreases with regular supplementation.

- **Vitamin C** has a laxative effect in very high doses, normally above 5g a day. Some people are very sensitive, even at 1g a day, while others can tolerate 10g a day. The ideal dose is the 'bowel tolerance' level so adjust your intake accordingly.

◆ VALUE FOR MONEY

For a supplement to be good value it must be well made, well formulated and reasonably priced. The quality of manufacture is hard to assess unless you have an advanced chemistry laboratory in your back room! However, there are four simple tests you can apply:

1. Are the stated number of tablets actually in the bottle? (We tested one company and found an average of 95 tablets instead of 100!)

2. Is the tablet coated all round and therefore easy to swallow? (Uncoated or badly coated tablets can break up or taste unpleasant.)

3. Does the label tell you everything you need to know? (The better the company, the more information they will give you.)

4. Does the company emphasise their quality control and, if asked, can they supply you with independent analyses of their products?

How Much is Safe?

J ust how safe are supplements? What happens if you take more vitamins or minerals than you need? How much is too much? These are common concerns, fuelled by media reports linking vitamin C with kidney stones and warnings against vitamin A in pregnancy. How much is fact and how much is fiction?

The optimal intake of a nutrient varies considerably for each individual, depending on their age, sex, health and numerous other factors. Therefore it is to be expected that the level of a vitamin that can induce signs of toxicity also varies considerably. During an illness, a person's need for a vitamin can increase dramatically. Vitamin C is the prime example of this – when a person is fighting an infection his or her requirements are much higher. In this chapter I have erred on the side of caution by listing the levels of nutrients that may induce toxicity in a small percentage of people, if taken over a short period of time (up to one month), and over a long period of time (three months to three years). I have also indicated which symptoms persist and which go away once the high level is reduced.

It's important to realise that just about everything is toxic if the dose is high enough. In 1990 a man died from drinking 10 litres of water in two hours. The greatest risk from the drug Ecstasy, say doctors from the Western General Hospital in Edinburgh, is not the drug itself but the risk of overdosing on water to stave off the side-effects of the drug. One user died from drinking too much water to combat dehydration. So the critical question is, how much more of the substance than is normally consumed would you have to take to reach toxic levels? In other words, what is the safety margin?

◆ THE SAFETY OF VITAMINS

The general conclusion, from a survey of the results of over 100 research papers in scientific journals, is that, for the majority of vitamins, with the exception of vitamins A and D, levels 100 times greater than the US RDA are likely to be safe for long-term ingestion. In practical terms, this means that you are extremely unlikely to have a toxic reaction to even the higher-dose supplements available in healthfood shops, unless you take a considerably greater number of tablets than recommended. This is broadly consistent with the public health record of deaths attributed to nutritional supplements. For example, a survey of Local Poison Control Centers in the US between the years 1983 and 1987 listed 1182 fatalities resulting from pharmaceutical drugs, and not one fatality resulting from a vitamin supplement. In Britain, I have been unable to find any death attributable to vitamin supplementation (as compared to approximately 15,000 deaths per year attributed to pharmaceutical drugs).

VITAMIN A

Vitamin A comes in two forms: the animal form, retinol, which is stored in the body; and the vegetable form, beta-carotene, which is converted into retinol, unless body levels are already high. Beta-carotene is therefore not considered toxic, although excessive intake can cause a reversible yellowing of the skin.

There are a number of incidences of adverse reactions to retinol, usually from intakes of 500,000iu or more, over a considerable length of time. The symptoms include peeling and redness of the skin, disturbed hair growth, lack of appetite and vomiting. According to Dr John Marks, director of medical studies at Girton College, Cambridge, 'Toxic reactions have been extremely rare below 30,000iu ... daily administration in adults up to about 50,000iu would appear to be safe.' This is consistent with estimates of the intake of 40,000iu of vitamin A that our ancestors would have eaten in a more tropical environment, although a large part of this would have come from beta-carotene.

A number of cases of toxicity and birth defects have been reported for a synthetic relative of vitamin A, isotretinoin, sold as the drug Roaccutane. These reports of birth defects have been wrongly extended to natural vitamin A. Five cases of birth defects have been reported in women taking large amounts of retinol (25,000 to 500,000iu per day). However, no clear cause and effect relationship has ever been established in any of these cases.

Other studies have shown that women who supplement their diet with multivitamins including vitamin A, usually at a level of 7500–25,000iu, have a lower incidence of birth defects. One study found a possible association. This study involved 22,747 women, of whom 121 gave birth to children with the kind of defect associated with, among other things, vitamin A toxicity. Of these 121, two of the cases could have been attributable to supplementing in excess of 10,000iu of vitamin A in the form of retinol. In view of the possibility that retinol, in large amounts, could induce birth defects, it is wise for women of child-bearing age to supplement no more than 10,000iu of retinol. The same caution does not apply to beta-carotene.

VITAMIN D

Of all the vitamins, vitamin D is the most likely to cause toxic reactions. Vitamin D encourages calcium absorption, and excessive intake can lead to calcification of soft tissue. However, the levels that create this effect are certainly in excess of 10,000iu and probably more like 50,000iu. A daily intake not exceeding 2000iu for adults and 1000iu for children is generally considered to be safe.

VITAMIN E

Vitamin E has been well researched for toxicity. A review of 216 trials of high-dose vitamin E in 10,000 patients showed that daily doses of 3000iu for up to 11 years, and 55,000iu for a few months, had no detrimental effect. However, adverse reactions have occasionally been reported at lower levels of 2000iu, especially in children, possibly due to an allergic reaction to the source of the vitamin E.

Vitamin E appears to enhance the anti-clotting effects of the drug Warfarin, so high levels are not recommended for people taking that drug. High levels are also best avoided by those suffering from rheumatic fever. Some old reports that vitamin

E should not be supplemented by women with breast cancer are inaccurate – it is actually highly beneficial to supplement in this condition. A daily intake of up to 1500iu is considered safe.

Vitamin C

Vitamin C is water-soluble so any excess is readily excreted from the body via the urine. RDAs vary considerably from country to country. A general consensus, based on up-to-date research, is that 100mg a day represents a good basic intake. The optimal intake is between 1000 and 3000mg a day.

A number of studies have investigated the effects of vitamin C on specific diseases, using over 10,000mg a day. The recommendation of these high levels has attracted controversy and allegations that vitamin C can cause kidney stone formation, interfere with B12 absorption, and cause a 'rebound scurvy' when supplementation is stopped. All these allegations have been shown to be without substance. The only problem with taking large amounts of vitamin C is that it can have a laxative effect. Generally, supplementing up to 5000mg of vitamin C can be considered safe.

B vitamins

B vitamins are water-soluble so any excess is readily excreted from the body via the urine. Thiamin (B1), riboflavin (B2), pantothenic acid (B5), B12 and biotin show no sign of toxicity at levels of at least 100 times the US RDA. Vitamin B3, in the form of niacin, causes a blushing sensation at levels of 75mg or more. This is part of its natural action and is not therefore generally considered to be a toxic effect.

According to Dr John Marks, director of medical studies at Girton College, Cambridge, 'doses of 200mg to 10g daily have been used therapeutically to lower blood cholesterol levels under medical control for periods of up to ten years or more, and though some reactions have occurred at these very high dosages, they have rapidly responded to cessation of therapy, and have often cleared even when therapy has been continued'. Levels of up to 2000mg per day on a continuous basis are considered safe, although they will induce blushing (vasodilation).

Vitamin B6 has been extensively tested for toxicity by a number of research groups, including the US government Food and Drug Administration who concluded, 'in man, side-effects were not encountered with daily administration of 50–200mg over periods of months'. Most of the unfounded reports of low-dose B6 causing nerve damage appear to be based on one well-documented case of a woman who increased her B6 intake from supplements from 500mg to 5000mg over a period of two years, and developed muscle weakness and pain, attributed to nerve damage.

One researcher, investigating seven cases of people taking 2000–5000mg a day of B6 for considerable lengths of time said that 'substantial improvement occurred in all cases in the months after withdrawal of pyridoxine, usually with improvement in gait and less discomfort in the extremities, but in some patients, residual neurological discomfort remained'. In rats, daily doses of 600mg/kg (equivalent to 38,000mg a day in a 10-stone person), by injection, caused peripheral neuropathy. Deficiency of vitamin B6 induces the same symptoms. The likely explanation for this is that pyridoxine, in order to become active in the body, where it helps enzymes to work, must be converted to pyridoxal-5-phosphate. If the body becomes saturated with excessive amounts of pyridoxine, this conversion doesn't take place, enzymes become saturated with simple pyridoxine and therefore don't work properly. In other words, a B6 excess may effectively induce B6 deficiency symptoms.

Since zinc is required for the conversion of pyridoxine to pyridoxal-5-phosphate, taking B6 with zinc is likely to reduce its toxicity. In any event, a daily intake of up to 200mg on a continuous basis is generally considered safe.

◆ THE SAFETY OF MINERALS

The safety of minerals depends on three factors. Firstly, the amount – all minerals show toxicity at exceedingly high doses. Secondly, the form – trivalent chromium, for example, is essential, while hexavalent chromium (which is not found in food or supplements) is very toxic. Thirdly, the balance with other minerals in the diet – iron supplementation, for instance, can exacerbate zinc deficiency since it is a zinc antagonist. The reason for this antagonism is that many minerals are atomically very similar to each other. So if you lack one mineral but take in an excess of another similar mineral it can slot into the wrong enzyme, speeding up or slowing down or simply stopping the enzyme from working.

In view of these factors, the levels given below as safe for long-term ingestion presuppose that other essential minerals are also adequately supplied. Larger amounts than those stated may also be safe for short-term ingestion, particularly for people with certain illnesses which increase the need for a particular mineral. Selenium requirement, for example, is thought to increase in certain types of cancer.

CALCIUM

Calcium comes in many forms, the best absorbed of which include calcium ascorbate, amino acid chelate, gluconate, orotate and carbonate. In normal, healthy people there is little danger of toxicity since the body excretes excessive amounts. Some cultures consume in excess of 2g a day from diet alone, so this amount is certainly considered safe. A dose of 3.6g per day is used to treat calcium deficiency disorders.

Problems of excessive calcium arise from other factors, such as excessive vitamin D intake (above 25,000iu per day), parathyroid or kidney disorders. Calcium interacts with magnesium and phosphorus. Calcium supplements should therefore only be taken by people who have an adequate magnesium and phosphorus intake, or who are also supplementing these elements. Phosphorus deficiency is rare, while magnesium deficiency is quite common. The ideal calcium/phosphorus ratio is probably 2:1. Less than 1:2 is not desirable. The ideal calcium/magnesium ratio is probably 3:2.

MAGNESIUM

Magnesium comes in many forms, the best absorbed of which include magnesium aspartate, amino acid chelate, gluconate, orotate and carbonate. Toxic effects of magnesium include flushing of the skin, thirst, low blood pressure, loss of reflexes and respiratory depression. Toxicity from taking supplements is only likely to occur in people with kidney disease. For normal, healthy adults a daily intake of up to 1000mg is considered safe. Magnesium interacts with calcium, so magnesium supplements should only be given to those with adequate calcium intake, or those supplementing calcium. The ideal magnesium/calcium ratio is probably 2:3 and, in cases of magnesium deficiency, 1:1.

IRON

Iron is one of the minerals that people are most frequently deficient in. At least 6 per cent of women in the UK get below the RDA from their diets. Iron comes in many different forms, the best absorbed of which include ferrous aspartate, amino acid chelate, succinate, lactate and gluconate. Ferric forms of iron are less well absorbed. Ferrous sulphate induces symptoms of toxicity in animals at lower levels than these forms. As little as 3g of ferrous sulphate can cause death in an infant, compared to 12g for an adult. Therefore supplements containing a significant amount of iron should be kept in a childproof container away from children.

Iron is stored in the body, so toxicity can result from chronic over-intake, producing haemosiderosis (a generalised deposition of iron within body tissue) or haemochromatosis (normally a hereditary condition resulting in cirrhosis of the liver, bronze pigmentation of the skin, diabetes, arthritis and heart abnormalities). Both conditions are extremely rare as a result of dietary intake. Up to 50mg a day is generally considered safe.

Iron is antagonistic to many other trace minerals including zinc, which is also commonly deficient, especially among pregnant and lactating women. So extra iron should not be supplemented without ensuring adequate zinc status or supplementing zinc. The normal requirement for zinc and iron is approximately equal.

ZINC

Zinc is one of the most thoroughly researched and widely deficient minerals. About a thousand papers are published each year indicating its value for a variety of conditions. The best absorbed forms of zinc include zinc picolinate, amino acid chelate, citrate and gluconate. Zinc supplementation is relatively non-toxic. In doses of 2000mg symptoms of nausea, vomiting, fever and severe anaemia have been reported. Small amounts of zinc, particularly in the form of zinc sulphate, can act as an irritant in the digestive tract when taken on an empty stomach. There is also some evidence that zinc, at levels of 300mg per day, may impair rather than improve immune function. It is generally considered safe to supplement up to 50mg per day.

Zinc is an iron, manganese and copper antagonist, so an adequate intake of these minerals is recommended if large amounts of zinc are taken over a long period of time. Manganese is very poorly absorbed. It is therefore generally advisable to supplement half as much manganese as zinc if more than 20mg of zinc is supplemented per day. The normal requirement for zinc is about ten times that of copper. Since the average intake of copper for those on a healthy diet is in the order of 2mg, those supplementing more than 20mg of zinc may be advised to add 1mg of copper for each additional 10mg of zinc. It is also best to ensure that at least 12mg of iron is supplemented when taking more than 20mg of zinc.

COPPER

Copper deficiency is quite rare, probably because we receive it from drinking water as well as from unrefined foods. The best absorbed forms of copper include copper amino acid chelate and gluconate. Requirements are low (2mg per day) and only 5mg a day is required to correct deficiency. Copper toxicity does occur, mainly due to excessive intake as a result of copper plumbing. Copper is also a strong antagonist of zinc, and for this reason it is not advisable to supplement more than 2mg or a tenth of one's intake of zinc. Copper also depletes manganese.

MANGANESE

Only 2–5 per cent of dietary manganese is absorbed, so larger dietary intakes have a small effect on overall body levels. The best forms for absorption include amino acid chelates, gluconates and orotates. There is some evidence that vitamin C may help the absorption of manganese. In animals it has been shown to be one of the least toxic of all trace elements. Toxicity has never been reported in man. A daily intake of up to 50mg is considered safe. Excessive zinc or copper intake interferes with manganese absorption.

SELENIUM

Selenium is required in very small amounts of 25–200mcg per day. It comes in two forms: organic such as selenomethionine or selenocystine, sometimes in the form of selenium yeast; and inorganic sodium selenite. The inorganic form is more toxic – toxicity occurs at levels of 1000mcg or more. The organic forms show toxicity above 2000mcg. No toxicity has been reported with either form at intakes of up to 750mcg. An intake of up to 500mcg for an adult is generally considered safe. In view of the relatively small difference between a beneficial and a detrimental intake, selenium should also be kept out of reach of children.

CHROMIUM

Chromium is found in two forms in nature – hexavalent and trivalent. Hexavalent chromium is much more toxic. However, it is not found in food or supplements so contamination can only occur from occupational exposure. Trivalent chromium has very low toxicity, partly because so little is absorbed. The best-absorbed forms of chromium are picolinate and amino acid chelate. Cats show signs of toxicity at 1000mg per day. An intake of up to 500mcg is certainly considered safe.

◆ THE SAFETY OF HERBAL REMEDIES

There are good grounds for being more cautious about herbal remedies. Many are not nutrients as such and may contain compounds that exert powerful effects on the body's chemistry. More is not necessarily better. Therefore it is wise not to exceed the stated dose for herbs and it is best to visit a qualified herbalist for a comprehensive recommendation. However, as far as I am aware, there are no reports of cat's claw or echinacea being toxic even when used at levels considerably above the recommended doses.

References

PART 1

1. *The Vitamin Controversy*, ION Press (1987); available from ION, £2.95.
Bateman Catering Organisation, 'A Square Meal for Britain?' (1981).
Queen Elizabeth College, University of London, *The Booker Health Report*,
Booker Health Foods (1985).
'Vitamin Scandal – Government Survey Reveals', *Optimum Nutrition*, 7.3
(4) (1994); available from ION, yearly subscription £9 for three maga-
zines.
2. Stephens et al, *Lancet*, vol 347 (23 March 1996).
3. Hemila, H. and Herman, Z.S., 'Vitamin C and the Common Cold: A
Retrospective Analysis of Chalmers' Review', *J Am. College Nutrition*, vol
14 (2) (1995), pp. 116–23.
4. Enstrom, J. and Pauling, L., 'Mortality among health-conscious elderly
Californians', *Proc. Natl. Acad. Sci.*, vol 79 (1982), pp. 6023–7.
5. Cheraskin, E. and Ringsdorf, 'Establishing a Suggested Optimum
Nutrition Allowance (SONA)' and 'What is Optimum?', *Optimum
Nutrition*, vol 7 (2) (1994), pp. 46–7.
6. *The Vitamin Controversy*, op. cit.
7. Davies, S., 'The Myth of the Balanced Diet', Power of Prevention
Conference (1993); available from ION – cassette 'T16 – The Myth of the
Balanced Diet', £5.95.
8. Hemila, 'Vitamin' C and the Common Cold'.

9. Chandra, R.K., 'Study of Multivitamin/mineral Supplementation in Elderly', *Lancet*, vol 340 (8828) (1992), pp. 1124–7.

10. Milunsky, A., 'Multivitamin/Folic acid Supplementation in Early Pregnancy Reduces the Prevalence of Neural Tube Defects', *JAMA*, vol 262 (20), (24 November 1989), pp. 2847–52.

11. Benton, D. and Roberts, G., 'Effect of Vitamin and Mineral Supplementation on Intelligence of a Sample of School Children', *Lancet* (23 January 1988).

12. Oakley, G., 'Eat Right and Take a Multivitamin', *New Engl J Med*, vol 338 (15) (9 April 1998), pp. 1060–1.

13. Colgan, M., *Your Personal Vitamin Profile*, Blond & Briggs (1983).

14. Mervyn, L., 'Mineral Losses in Refined Food', unpublished research.

15. 'What's Cooking?', Reprint No. 61, obtainable by phoning ION, London, UK Tel: 020 8877 9993.

16. Crawford, M. and Marsh, D., *Nutrition and Evolution – The Driving Force*, Keats, Connecticut USA (1995).

17. Cheraskin, E., *Vitamin C – Who Needs It?*, Arlington Press, Alabama USA (1993).

18. East Anglian Cancer Intelligence Unit, Dept. of Community Medicine, University of Cambridge, *Report of Cancer Incidence and Projections for Macmillan Cancer Relief* (June 1977).

19. Davies, S., 'Scientific and Ethical Foundations of Nutritional Medicine. Part 1 – Evolution, Adaptation and Health', *J Nut Med*, vol 2 (1991), p. 3.

20. Ash, J., 'Investigation into the Mechanisms of the Effects of Azo Dyes on Hyperactive Children', Final year project, School of Biological Sciences, University of Surrey, Guildford, UK; copy held by Dr Neil Ward.

21. Patterson, C., 'An Alternative Perspective – Lead Pollution in the Environment', in *Lead in the Human Environment*, Commission of Natural Resources Research Council, Washington DC, National Academy of Sciences (1980), pp. 265–349.

PART 2

1. Bryce-Smith, D., 'Boron: Candidate for Essentiality', *Felmore Newsletter*, 151.

2. Chazin, S., 'Is iron a danger in your diet?' *Reader's Digest* (December 1995).

3. Ibid.

4. Harland, B.F. and Harden-Williams, B.A., 'Is vanadium of human nutritional importance yet?' *J Am Diet Assoc*, vol 94 (1993), pp. 891–4.

5. Brichard, S.M. and Henguin, J.C., 'The role of vanadium in the management of diabetes', *Trends Pharmacol Sci*, vol 16 (1995), pp. 265–70.

6. Wunderlich, R., *Sugar and Your Health*, Good Health Publications, Florida (1982).

7. Davies, S., 'Zinc, Nutrition and Health', chapter in *1984/5 Yearbook of Nutritional Medicine* (1985).

8. Davies, S., et al., 'Age-related decreases in chromium levels in 51,665 hair, sweat and serum samples from 40,872 patients – implications for the prevention of cardiovascular disease and type II diabetes mellitus', *Metabolism*, vol 46(5) (1997), pp. 1–4.

9. Morris, B., et al., 'Correlations between abnormalities in chromium and glucose metabolism in a group of diabetics', *Clin Chem*, vol 34 (1988), pp. 1525–6.

Urberg, M., et al., 'Hypocholesterolemic effects of nicotinic acid and chromium supplementation', *Fam Pract*, vol 27 (1988), pp. 603–6 .

10. Riales, R., et al., 'Effects of chromium chloride supplementation on glucose tolerance and serium lipids including high density lipoprotein of adult men', *Am J Clin Nutr*, vol 34 (1981), pp. 2670–8.

Abraham, A., et al., 'The effects of chromium supplementation on serum glucose and lipids in patients with and without non-insulin-dependent diabetes', *Metabolism*, vol 41 (1992), p. 768.

11. Salonen, J.T., et al., 'Risk of cancer in relation to serum concentrations of selenium and vitamins A and E', *BMJ*, vol 290 (1985), pp. 417–20.

12. *Am J Clin Nutr*, vol 64 (1966), pp. 190–6 .

13. *Cancer Epidemiol Biomarkers Prevention*, vol 6(10) (1977), pp. 769–74.

14. Yong, L-C, et al., 'Intakes of vitamins E, C and A and risk of lung cancer: the NHANES I epidemiologic follow-up study', *Am J Epidemiol*, vol 146(3) (1997), pp. 231–43.

15. Shklar, G., et al., 'The effectiveness of a mixture of beta-carotene, alpha-tocopherol and ascorbic acid for cancer prevention', *Nutrition and Cancer*, vol 20(2) (1993).

16. Aaman, Z., et al., 'Plasma concentrations of vitamins A and E and carotenoids in Alzheimer's Disease', *Age and Aging*, vol 21(2) (1992), pp. 91–4.

17. Jacques, P.F., 'Relationship of vitamin C status to cholesterol and blood pressure', *Ann NY Acad Sci*, vol 669 (1992), pp. 205–14.

18. Robertson, J.M., et al., 'Vitamin E intake and risk of cataracts in humans', *Ann NY Acad Sci*, vol 570 (1989), pp. 372–82.

19. Bond, G., et al., 'Dietary vitamin A and lung cancer: results of a case-control study among chemical workers', *Nutrition and Cancer*, vol 9(2) (1987), pp. 109–21.

20. Mayne, S.T., 'Dietary beta-carotene and lung cancer risk in U.S. non-smokers', *J Nat Cancer Inst*, vol 86(1) (1994), pp. 33–8.

21. Garwal, H.S., et al., 'Response of oral leukoplakia to beta-carotene', *J Clin Oncology*, vol 8 (1990), pp. 1715–20.

22. Manson, J.E., et al., 'A prospective study of antioxidant vitamins and incidence of coronary heart disease in women', *Circulation*, vol 84(4) (1991), pp. 115–46.

23. Osilesi, O., et al., 'Blood pressure and plasma lipids during ascorbic acid supplementation in borderline hypertensive and normotensive adults', *Nutr Research*, vol 11 (1991), pp. 405–12.

24. Folkers, K., et al., 'Relevance of the biosynthesis of coenzyme Q10 and of the four bases of DNA as a rationale for the molecular causes of cancer and a therapy', *Biochem Biophys Res Commun*, vol 224(2) (1996), pp. 358–61.

Folkers, K., et al., 'Activities of vitamin Q10 in animal models and a serious deficiency in patients with cancer', *Biochem Biophys Res Commun*, vol 234(2) (1997), pp. 296–9.

25. Lockwood, K., et al., 'Progress on therapy of breast cancer with vitamin Q10 and the regression of metastases', *Biochem Biophys Res Commun*, vol 212(1) (1995), pp. 172–7.

26. Lockwood, K., et al., 'Apparent partial remission of breast cancer in "high risk" patients supplemented with nutritional antioxidants, essential fatty acids and coenzyme Q10', *Mol Aspects Med*, vol 15S (1994), pp. S231–S240 .

27. Kidd, P.M., 'Glutathione: systemic protectant against oxidative and free radical damage', *Alt Med Rev*, vol 2(3) (1997), pp. 155–75.

28. Donnerstag, B., et al., 'Reduced glutathione and s-acetylglutathione as selective apoptosis-inducing agents in cancer therapy', *Cancer Letters*, vol 110 (1996), pp. 63–70.

29. Ohlenschlagen, G. and Treusch, G., 'Reduced glutathione and antho-cyans – redox recycling and redox recycling in biological systems', *Praxis-telegramm*.

30. Garcia-Giralt, E., et al., 'Preliminary study of GSH I-cysteine antho-cyane (Reconstat Compositum ™) in metastatic colorectal carcinoma with relative denutrition', Seventh International Congress on Anti-Cancer Treatment (February 1997).

31. Masquelier, J., *J Medicinal Plant Res*, vol 7 (1980), pp. 243–56.

32. Becker, Y., et al., *Connect Tissue Res*, vol 8 (1981), p. 77.

33. Fuchs, J., et al., 'Studies on kipoate effects on blood redox state in human immunodeficiency virus infected patients', *Arzneim Forsch*, vol 43 (1993), pp. 1359–62.

34. Chandra, R., 'Effect of vitamin and trace element supplementation on immune responses and infection in elderly subjects', *Lancet*, vol 340 (1992), pp. 1124–7.

35. Harakeh, S., et al., 'Suppression of human immunodeficiency virus replication by ascorbate in chronically and acute infected cells', *Proc Natl Acad Sci*, vol 87 (1990), pp. 245–9.

36. Godfrey, J., et al., 'Zinc for treating the common cold: review of all clinical trials since 1984', *Altern Ther*, vol 2(6) (1996), pp. 63–72.

37. *Br J Phytotherapy*, vol 2 (1991), p. 2.

38. Roesler, J., et al., 'Application of purified polysaccharides from cell cultures of the plant *Echinacea purpurea* to mice mediates protection against systemic infections with *Listeria monocytogenes* and *Candida albicans*', *Intl J Immunopharmac*, vol 13 (1991), pp. 27–37.

39. Erhard, M., et al., 'Effect of Echinacea, Aconitum, Lachesis and Apis extracts and their combinations on phagocytosis of human granulocytes', *Phytotherapy Res*, vol 8 (1994), pp. 14–17.

40. Zakay-Jones, Z., et al., 'Inhibition of several strains of influenza virus *in vitro* and reduction of symptoms by an elderberry extract (*Sambucus nigra L.*) during an outbreak of influenza B panama', *Alt Comp Med*, vol 1, (1995), pp. 361–9.

41. Benton, D., 'Effect of vitamin and mineral supplementation on intelligence of a sample of school children', *Lancet* (23 January 1988).

42. Dean, W. and Morgenthaler, J., *Smart Drugs and Nutrients*, B&J Publications (1990).

43. Pilch, H., et al., 'Piracetam elevates muscarinic cholinergic receptor density in the frontal cortex of aged but not of young mice', *Psychopharmacology*, vol 94 (1988), pp. 74–8.

44. Stoll, A.L., et al., 'Omega 3 fatty acids in bipolar disorder', *Arch Gen Psychiatry*, vol 56 (1999), p. 407.

45. Stordy, B.J., 'Benefit of docosahexaenoic acid supplements of dark

adaptation in dyslexics', *Lancet*, vol 346 (1995), p. 385.

46. Allard, M., 'Treatment of old age disorders with Gingko biloba extract', *La Presse Medicale*, vol 15(31) (1986), p. 1540.

Hindmarch, I., 'Activity of Gingko biloba extract on short-term memory', *La Presse Medicale*, vol 15(31) (1986), pp. 1562–92.

47. Funfgeld, E., 'A natural and broad spectrum nootropic substance for treatment of SDAT – the Gingko biloba extract', *Progress in Clinical and Biological Research*, vol 317 (1989), pp. 1247–60.

48. Loriaux, S., et al., 'The effects of nicotinic acid (niacin) and xanthinol nicotinate on human memory on different categories of age, a double blind study', *Psychopharmacology*, vol 87 (1985), pp. 390–5.

49. Pearson, D. and Shaw, S., *Life Extension: A Practical Scientific Approach*, Warner Books, New York (1982).

50. Stewart, J.W., et al., 'Low B6 levels in depressed outpatients', *Biol Psychiat.*, vol 141 (1982), pp. 271–2.

51. Poldinger, et al., 'A functional-dimensional approach to depression: serotonin deficiency and target syndrome in a comparison of 5-hydroxytryptophan and fluvoxamine', *Psychopathology*, vol 24 (1991), pp. 53–81.

52. Miller, A., *Alternative Medicine Review*, vol 3(1) (1998).

53. Beckman, N., 'Phytoestrogens and compounds that affect estrogen metabolism – part 2', *Aust J Med Herbalism*, vol 7(2) (1995), pp. 27–33.

54. Messina M. and Messina V., 'Increasing use of soy foods and their potential roles in cancer prevention', *Perspectives in Practice*, vol 91(7) (1991), pp. 836–40.

55. Dwyer, J., et al., 'Tofu and soy drinks contain phyto-oestrogens', *J M Diet Assoc*, vol 94(7) (1994), pp. 739–43.

56. Dittmar, F., et al., 'Premenstrual syndrome: treatment with a phytopharmaceutical', *TW Gnakol*, vol 5(1) (1992), pp. 60–8.

57. Dittmar, F., *Out of the Earth*, Viking, Penguin (1991).

58. Kremer, et al., *Arth & Rheum*, vol 33(6) (1989), pp. 729–33.

59. Kremer, et al., *Lancet,* vol 1 (1985), pp. 184–7.

60. Sperling, *Med World News* (14 July 1986).

61. 'Curcuminoids – the active principles from turmeric root', *Sabinsa Corporation*.

62. Joe, B., et al., 'Effect on curcumin and capsaicin on arachidonic acid metabolism and lysosomal enzyme secretion by rat peritoneal macrophages', *Lipids*, vol 32(11) (1997), pp. 1173–80.

63. Singh, G.G., et al., 'New phytotherapeutic agent for treatment of

arthritis and allied disorders with novel mode of action', IV International Congress on Phytotherapy, Munich, Germany Abstract SL74.

64. Gupta, V., et al., 'Chemistry and pharmacology of gum resin of Boswellia Serrata', *Indian Drugs*, vol 24(5) (1986), pp. 221–31.

65. Kulkarni, R., et al., 'Treatment of oesteoarthritis with a herbal formulation: a double-blind, placebo controlled, crossover study', *J Ethnopharm*, vol 33 (1991), pp. 91–5; see also same author, *Ind J Pharm*, vol 24 (1992), pp. 98–101.

66. Jacob, Stanley MD, Lawrence, Ronald MD PhD and Zucker, Martin, *The Miracle of MSM, The Natural Solution for Pain*, Putnam (1999).

67. Kiuchi, F., et al., 'Inhibition of prostaglandin and leukotriene biosynthesis by gingerols and diarylheptanoids', *Chem Pharm Bull*, vol 40 (1992), pp. 387–91.

68. Srivastava, K.C. and Mustafa, T., 'Ginger (*Zingiber officianale*) and rheumatic disorders', *Med Hypothesis*, vol 39 (1992), pp. 342–8.

69. Negre-Salvayre, A., et al., 'Additional antilipoperoxidant activities of alpha-tocopherol and ascorbic acid on membrane-like systems are potentiated by rutin', *Pharmacol*, vol 42 (1991), pp. 262–72.

70. Lindahl, M., 'Flavonoids as phospholipase A2 inhibitors: importance of their structure for selective inhibition of group II phospholipase A2', *Inflammation*, vol 21(3) (1997), pp. 347–56.

71. Gordon, 'New dimensions in calcium metabolism', *Osteopathic Annals* (1982).

72. Mankin, *Orthop Clin North Am*, vol 2 (1972), p. 19.

73. NASA report, American Medical Association Symposium, Florida (1982).

Korcak, M., *J Am Med Assoc*, vol 247 (1982), p. 8.

74. Marier, J.R., 'Magnesium content of the food supply in the modern-day world', *Magnesium*, vol 5(1) (1986), pp. 1–8.

75. Loughead, et al., 'A role for magnesium in neonatal parathyroid gland function', *J Am Coll Nutr*, vol 10(2) (1991), pp. 123–6.

76. Hamilton and Minski, *Sci Total Environ*, vol 1 (1972/3), p. 375.

77. Abraham, Dr G., *J Nut Med*, vol 2 (1991), pp. 165–78.

78. Herzberg, M., et al., 'The effect of estrogen replacement therapy on zinc in serum and urine', *Ostet Gynecol*, vol 87(6) (1996), pp. 1035–40.

79. Neilson, et al., *FASEB J*, vol 1 (1987), p. 394.

80. Germano, C., *The Osteoporosis Solution*, Kensington Books (1999).

81. Thomas, M., et al., *New Engl. J Med*, vol 338 (1998), pp. 777–83.

82. Karzel, K. and Lee, K.J., 'Effect of hexosamine derivatives on

mesenchymal metabolic processes of *in vitro* cultured fetal bone explants', *Z Rheumatol*, vol 41 (1982), pp. 212–18.

Setnikar, I., et al., 'Antireactive properties of glucosamine sulfate', *Arzneim Forsch*, vol 41 (1991), pp. 157–61.

83. Setnikar, I., et al., 'Pharmacokinetics of glucosamine in the dog and in man', *Arzneim Forsch*, vol 36 (1986), pp. 729–33.

84. Hehne, H.J., et al., 'Therapy of gonarthrosis using chondroprotective substances. Prospective comparative study of glucosamine sulphate and glycosaminoglycan polysulphate', *Fortschr Med*, vol 102 (1984), pp. 676–82.

Recommended Reading

Cheraskin, E., *Vitamin C – Who Needs It?*, Arlington Press, Alabama, USA, 1993

Crawford, Professor Michael and Marsh, D., *Nutrition and Evolution – The Driving Force*, Keats Publishing, Connecticut, USA, 1995

Colgan, M., *Your Personal Vitamin Profile*, Blond & Briggs, 1983

Dean, W. and Morgenthaler, J., *Smart Drugs and Nutrients*, B & J Publications, 1990

Dittmar, F., *Out of the Earth*, Viking Penguin, 1991

Germano, C., *The Osteoporosis Solution*, Kensington Books, 1999

Holford, Patrick, *The Optimum Nutrition Bible*, Piatkus, 1997

Holford, Patrick, *Beat Stress and Fatigue*, Piatkus, 1999

Holford, Patrick, *Say No to Cancer*, Piatkus, 1999

Holford, Patrick, *Say No to Arthritis*, Piatkus, 1999

Holford, Patrick, *Improve Your Digestion*, Piatkus, 1999

Holford, Patrick and Meek, Jennifer, *Boost Your Immune System*, Piatkus, 1998

Holford, Patrick and Neil, Kate, *Balancing Hormones Naturally*, Piatkus, 1999

Holford, Patrick and Ridgway, Judy, *The Optimum Nutrition Cookbook*, Piatkus, 1999

ION, *The Vitamin Controversy*, ION, 1987; available from ION, £2.95

Jacob MD, S., Lawrence MD, R. and Zucker, M., *The Miracle of MSM, The Natural Solution for Pain*, Putnam, 1999

Pearson, D. and Shaw, S., *Life Extension: A Practical Scientific Approach*, Warner Books, New York, 1982

Wunderlich, R., *Sugar and Your Health*, Good Health Publications, Florida, 1982

Index

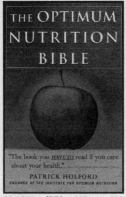
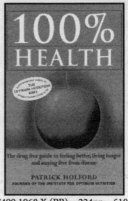
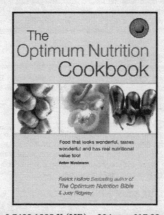
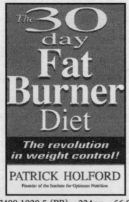
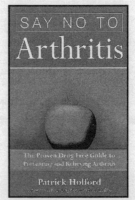